Vol. 33, Issue 6, December 2017

# Visceral Medicine

Gastroenterology, Endoscopy and Surgery –
The Interdisciplinary Approach to Gastrointestinal Disease

Focus

*Karl J. Oldhafer,* Hamburg
*Yuzo Yamamoto,* Akita
(Guest Editors)

## Frontiers of Liver Surgery

**Invited Articles**

**Interdisciplinary Discussion**



Further Sections

**Clinical Therapeutic Review**

**PharmaNews**

**Meetings and Conferences**

KARGER

Basel · Freiburg · Paris · London · New York · Chennai · New Delhi ·
Bangkok · Beijing · Shanghai · Tokyo · Kuala Lumpur · Singapore · Sydney

**Vol. 33, Issue 6, December 2017**

# Visceral Medicine

Gastroenterology, Endoscopy and Surgery – The Interdisciplinary Approach to Gastrointestinal Disease

Founded in 1984 as 'Chirurgische Gastroenterologie mit interdisziplinären Gesprächen' by A. Akovbiantz, H. Denk, K.-J. Paquet and C.E. Zöckler



**S. Karger GmbH**
P.O. Box, 79095 Freiburg, Germany

**Editorial Office**
Alexander Eitner
a.eitner@karger.com

Associated Organ for Continuing Education

KARGER

Basel · Freiburg · Paris · London · New York · Chennai · New Delhi · Bangkok · Beijing · Shanghai · Tokyo · Kuala Lumpur · Singapore · Sydney

KARGER

Basel · Freiburg · Paris · London · New York · Chennai · New Delhi · Bangkok · Beijing · Shanghai · Tokyo · Kuala Lumpur · Singapore · Sydney

Visceral Medicine

# Contents

Vol. 33, Issue 6, December 2017

## Focus: Frontiers of Liver Surgery

Guest Editors: Karl J. Oldhafer (Hamburg), Yuzo Yamamoto (Akita)



KARGER

Fax +49 761 4 52 07 14
Information@Karger.com
www.karger.com



Accessible online at:
www.karger.com/vis

Visceral Medicine

# Contents

**Vol. 33, Issue 6, December 2017**

Clinical Therapeutic Review



KARGER

Fax +49 761 4 52 07 14
Information@Karger.com
www.karger.com



Accessible online at:
www.karger.com/vis

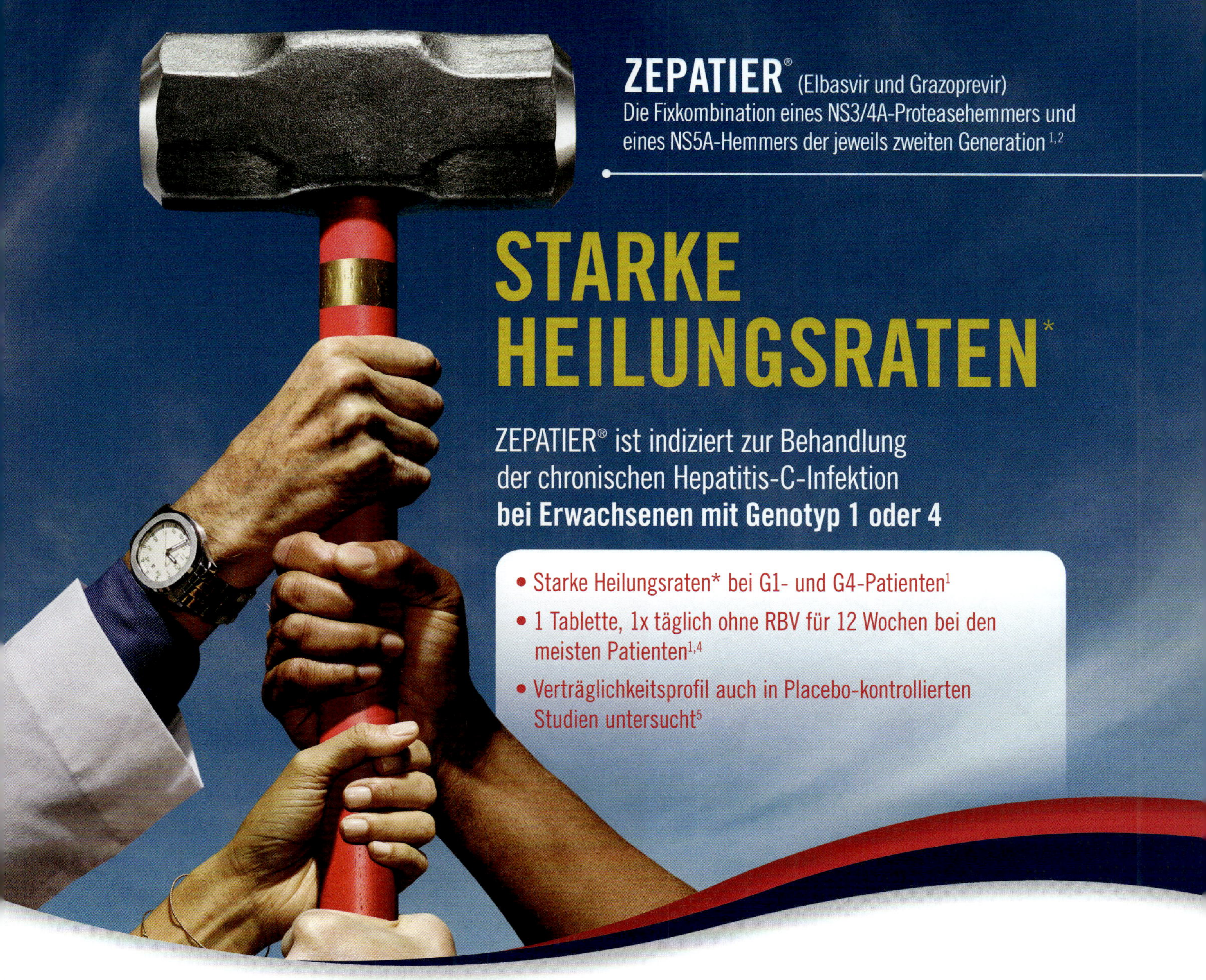




1. ZEPATIER® Fachinformation, Stand Juli 2017.
2. Clark VC, Peter JA, Nelson DR. New therapeutic strategies in HCV: second-generation protease inhibitors. Liver Int. 2013; 33(suppl 1): 80 – 84. doi:10.1111/liv.12061.
3. European Association for the Study of the Liver. Recommendations on Treatment of Hepatitis C 2015. J Hepatol. 2015; 63: 199 – 236.
4. Gower E., Estes C., Blach S., Razavi-Shearer K., Razavi H. Global epidemiology and genotype distribution of the hepatitis C virus infection. J Hepatol. 2014; 61: S45 – S57.
5. Dusheiko G. M., Manns M. P., Vierling J. M. et al. Safety and tolerability of elbasvir/grazoprevir in patients with chronic hepatitis C: an integrated analysis of phase 2 – 3 trials. Poster 712. Presented at: American Association for the Study of Liver Diseases Meeting; November 13 – 17, 2015; San Francisco, CA.

Visceral Medicine

Editorial

Visc Med 2017;33:405–406
DOI: 10.1159/000485169

Published online: December 5, 2017

# Frontiers of Liver Surgery

Yuzo Yamamoto[a] Karl J. Oldhafer[b,c]

[a] Department of Gastroenterological Surgery, Akita University Graduate School of Medicine, Akita, Japan;
[b] General and Visceral Surgery, Surgical Oncology, Asklepios Hospital Barmbek, Hamburg, Germany;
[c] Semmelweis Medical Faculty, Campus Hamburg, Hamburg, Germany

In the past, liver surgery has had key opportunities to undergo a dramatic evolution. These were supported by several innovative discoveries and inventions. The establishment of detailed knowledge of liver anatomy played a critical role in the development of liver surgery. As epoch-making events in anatomy, the discovery of the vasculo-biliary sheath (Francis Glisson, 1654), the definition of the right and left liver by Rex-Cantlie's line (Hugo Rex and James Cantlie, 1888 and 1889), the discovery of the hepatic venous system (Ton That Tung, 1939), as well as the identification of liver segments according to the portal system (Claude Couinaud, 1954) can be named. Regarding the aspect of surgical technique, cross-clamping of the hepatic pedicle (James Hogarth Pringle, 1908), preliminary vascular control (Jean-Louis Lortat-Jacob, 1952), and the finger fracture method (Tien-Yu Lin, 1960) formed the basis for the present procedures. This precise knowledge of anatomy and the corresponding techniques created modern liver surgery, e.g. anatomical subsegmentectomy (today called segmentectomy according to the IHPBA Brisbane 2000 nomenclature) in combination with ultrasound-guided dye injection (Masatoshi Makuuchi, 1984) and Glissonean approach (Ken Takasaki, 1990). Besides these developments, strategies to protect the function of liver remnant were described. In addition, total hepatic vascular exclusion under hypothermic perfusion (Joseph G. Fortner, 1974), ex-situ liver resection (Rudolf Pichlmayr, 1989), anterior approach (Kazue Ozawa, 1990), and liver hanging maneuver for anterior approach (Jacques Belghiti, 2001) were also noteworthy technical innovations.

Furthermore, developments in order to assess the hepatic functional reserve and to augment the volume of liver remnant largely contributed to the prevention of post-hepatectomy liver failure and thus to the safety of liver surgery. However, the most recent epoch-making innovation in liver surgery seems to be the ALPPS (associating liver partition and portal vein ligation for staged hepatectomy) procedure – initially introduced as 'in-situ split' liver resection – which made a vast impact in 2011. Since this procedure enables an astonishing increase of volume in the future liver remnant, it fascinated innovative surgeons immediately. However, as time for testing and improvement is required for every new technology, the ALPPS procedure must also undergo the process of evaluation and refinements as well as the analysis of its mechanism in order to find its proper place in the armamentarium of liver surgery, especially in relation to the already established portal vein embolization (PVE).

For this special topic of Visceral Medicine, we requested inventors of the ALPPS procedure [1] and of PVE [2] to disclose the behind-the-scenes story of invention in the light of a teaching by Confucius: 'Look for the old so as to learn the new' (fig. 1). These recounts may provide us with hints for overcoming the unresolved challenges. Additionally, we asked an expert radiologist of PVE as well as two driving forces of the ALPPS procedure in the world to contribute articles on the state-of-the-art technique of PVE to obtain an optimal hypertrophy of the liver [3], on the relationship between hypertrophy and liver function in ALPPS [4], and on the pitfalls in PVE and ALPPS [5]. Moreover, since the modalities of assessing the functional reserve of the liver differ between Western and Eastern countries, we asked two experts in the field from each area to delineate the currently most reliable methods [6, 7]. Finally, the Hamburg group summarized the impact of the first International ALPPS Expert Meeting 2015 [8].

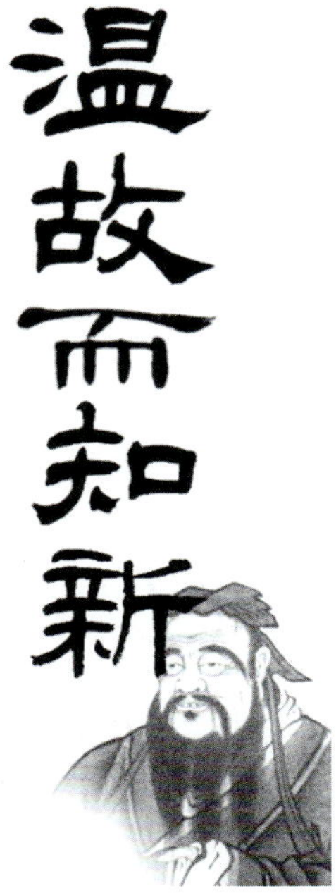


**Fig. 1.** 'Look for the old so as to learn the new' (teaching by Confucius).

When reading the articles of this special topic, you will easily recognize that there is still a slight difference in tone regarding the understanding of

KARGER

Fax +49 761 4 52 07 14
Information@Karger.com
www.karger.com



Accessible online at:
www.karger.com/vis

Yuzo Yamamoto, M.D., Ph.D.
Department of Gastroenterological Surgery
Akita University Graduate School of Medicine
1-1-1 Hondo, Akita 010-8543, Japan
yamamoto-kyt@umin.ac.jp

the features of the ALPPS procedure even among experts. While being someone who vehemently recommends various indications of the ALPPS procedure, Professor Schlitt, the inventor of ALPPS, humbly advises that such an invasive medical technology should be applied, with correct recognition of its absolute value and field of application, but not as a 'fashion of the times'. Thus, it can be well understood that liver surgeons carefully foster this new procedure while having a clear understanding of the risks and challenges involved. In contrast, there would be a need to internationally standardize the evaluation modalities of hepatic functional reserve in order to analyze the imbalance between the speed of volume increase and the speed of functional augmentation in ALPPS as well as in PVE, because international cooperation is absolutely necessary in the case of such a procedure which is not performed by many health professionals.

By means of this special topic, we are hoping that the readers correctly rate the values of ALPPS and PVE from the interdisciplinary viewpoint of expertise in surgery, internal medicine, radiology, oncology, and even pathophysiology. This will help in finding an answer regarding the proper area of application of these techniques without delay and result in a further favorable development. Consequently, liver surgery contributes to saving and extending the lives of many critically ill patients with advanced liver tumors.

Finally, the guest editors would like to express their sincere gratitude to the authors involved who provided such valuable contributions to this special topic on 'Frontiers of Liver Surgery'.

## References


1 Schlitt HJ, Hackl C, Lang SA: 'In-situ split' liver resection/ALPPS – historical development and current practice. Visc Med 2017;33:DOI: 10.1159/000479850.

2 Shinkawa H, Takemura S, Tanaka S, Kubo S: Portal vein embolization: history and current indications. Visc Med 2017;33:DOI: 10.1159/000479474.

3 Huang SY, Aloia TA: Portal vein embolization: state-of-the-art technique and options to improve liver hypertrophy. Visc Med 2017;33:DOI: 10.1159/000480034.

4 Kang D, Schadde E: Hypertrophy and liver function in ALPPS: correlation with morbidity and mortality. Visc Med 2017;33:DOI: 10.1159/000479477.

5 Schnitzbauer AA: A comparison of pitfalls after ALLPS stage 1 or portal vein embolization in small-for-size setting hepatectomies. Visc Med 2017;33:DOI: 10.1159/000480100.

6 Rassam F, Olthof PB, Bennink RJ, van Gulik TM: Current modalities for the assessment of future remnant liver function. Visc Med 2017;33:DOI: 10.1159/000480385.

7 Iimuro Y: ICG clearance test and 99mTc-GSA SPECT/CT fusion images. Visc Med 2017;33:DOI: 10.1159/000479046.

8 Stavrou GA, Donati M, Fard-Aghaie MH, Zeile M, Huber TM, Stang A, Oldhafer KJ: Did the International ALPPS Meeting 2015 have an impact on daily practice? The Hamburg Barmbek experience of 58 cases. Visc Med 2017;33:DOI: 10.1159/000479476.

Visceral Medicine

Review Article

Visc Med 2017;33:408–412
DOI: 10.1159/000479850

Published online: November 29, 2017

# 'In-Situ Split' Liver Resection/ALPPS – Historical Development and Current Practice

Hans J. Schlitt[a] Christina Hackl[a] Sven Arke Lang[a, b]

[a]Department of Surgery, University of Regensburg Medical Center, Regensburg, Germany;
[b]Department of Surgery, University of Freiburg, Freiburg i.Br., Germany

**Keywords**

Liver resection · Technique · In-situ split · ALPPS · Indication

**Summary**

**Background:** Liver tumors that are extensive, multifocal, or critically located frequently require advanced techniques of liver resection including 'functional augmentation' of liver segments. Here we describe the invention and stepwise establishment of a new technique – termed 'in-situ split' liver resection or 'ALPPS' – enabling liver resection in certain situations. **Methods:** The development of the technique in the first and the subsequent 8 patients in the index center, and also the method's spread throughout Germany and the world were reviewed. **Results:** In 2007, in the first patient, the new technique was developed intraoperatively by necessity. Due to the convincing outcome, it was deliberately applied again several months later in another patient, and thereafter (sparsely) used for liver resection for various indications. Following oral communication, the method spread throughout Germany, and later – mainly following the publication of the initial multicentric German series – very quickly disseminated worldwide. Currently, it is used for a very (if not overly) broad spectrum of indications by many hepatobiliary surgery centers. **Conclusion:** In-situ split/ALPPS is a newly developed technique for liver resection, which was established for very specific situations. This method has created a hype, and is currently used rather generously by many centers worldwide.



## Introduction

The limiting factor for (potentially curative) liver resection for certain primary or secondary tumors is the amount of functionally sufficient liver tissue that must remain [1]. If too small a left lateral section were to remain, preoperative embolization of the right portal vein, with or without embolization of the portal vein branches to liver segment IV, is an established technique [2]. However, the volume increase in the left lateral section is between 20 and 70% within approximately 6 weeks, i.e. highly variable and taking a rather long time [3, 4]. Moreover, in certain tumors, e.g. hilar cholangiocarcinoma (hCCC; Klatskin tumor), the preoperative embolization of the right side does no longer allow for an intraoperative strategy change to a left hepatectomy if required. Therefore, this approach is suboptimal in several situations. Moreover, it does not allow highly sensitive imaging of the left lateral section for the detection of small additional tumor load by intraoperative ultrasound (or even contrast-enhanced ultrasound) prior to deciding on the treatment strategy. Thus, a novel strategy was required to overcome these issues. The new technique, the development of which is described in this paper, is based on technical experience with both liver resection and in-situ split liver transplantation. This technique, termed 'in-situ split' liver resection and later found in the literature as ALPPS (associating liver partition and portal vein ligation for staged hepatectomy), was developed by the author by chance, and then started to conquer the hepato-pancreato-biliary (HPB) surgery world, first in Germany and then throughout the world. Here we describe the history of this development including details of the first case.

### *Patients*

The indications, perioperative considerations, as well as perioperative data of our first 9 patients were analyzed retrospectively. These patients underwent surgery between September 2007 and 2010. Details of the patients and procedures are given below.

KARGER

Fax +49 761 4 52 07 14
Information@Karger.com
www.karger.com



Accessible online at:
www.karger.com/vis

Prof. Dr. med. Hans J. Schlitt
Department of Surgery
University of Regensburg Medical Center
Franz-Josef-Strauß-Allee 11, 93053 Regensburg, Germany
hans.schlitt@ukr.de

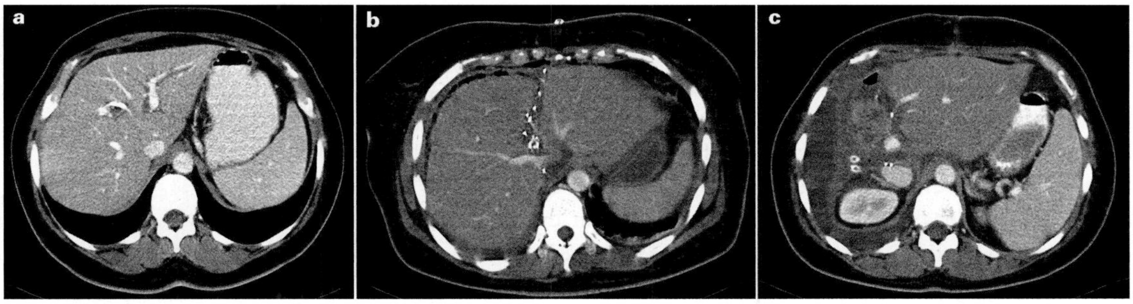


**Fig. 1.** First patient (hilar cholangiocarcinoma, Klatskin tumor) in whom an 'in-situ split' liver resection/ALPPS was performed in September 2007. **a** Contrast-enhanced computed tomography (CT) scan prior to the first surgery: dilated bile ducts, particularly in the left lateral section of the liver, in spite of preoperative drainage by endostent + percutaneous transhepatic cholangiography drainage (PTCD). **b** Contrast-enhanced CT scan 8 days after the first surgery with marked volume increase in the left lateral section. **c** Contrast-enhanced CT scan 7 day after the second surgery showing marked size increase of the remaining left lateral section.

*Methods*

In addition to the analysis of our patients, a non-systematic review of the literature as well as of conference reports and personal communications was performed to form the basis for the further assessment of the use of the novel technique.

## First Case of 'In-Situ Split' Liver Resection

A 49-year-old female patient presented with painless jaundice from suspected hCCC (Klatskin tumor) Bismuth type IV. Because of high serum bilirubin (15 mg/dl) with dilated bile ducts on both sides of the liver, a biliary stent was initially placed endoscopically to the right liver in a peripheral hospital, and the patient was then referred to our center. Upon admission, serum bilirubin was 5 mg/dl. After a review of all imaging results, it was decided to perform a right trisectionectomy after preoperative decompression of the left lateral ducts (fig. 1a). This could not be achieved via endoscopic retrograde cholangiography (ERC); therefore, a percutaneous transhepatic cholangiography and drainage (PTCD) was placed via the right side into the left ductal system. Bilirubin was 2 mg/dl, and surgery was performed on September 3, 2007. A preoperative volumetry had not been performed, and during surgery, the left lateral section was found to be too small (fig. 1a): retrospective volumetry showed 370 g with a patient body weight of 78 kg. Hence it was spontaneously decided during surgery to try and quickly induce hypertrophy of the left lateral section by de-portalizing the right liver while already performing the parenchymal dissection along the right side of the falciform ligament, thereby completely devascularizing segment IV in preparation for the final resection to be performed in a second step. Moreover, the left bile duct was divided at the base of the round ligament, about 2 cm away from the hepatic bifurcation, and a frozen section of the proximal bile duct resection margin was shown to be tumor-free. The bile duct towards the bifurcation was then suture-closed, and a Roux-en-Y hepaticojejunostomy was performed to the left duct. In order to facilitate the completion surgery, the right hepatic artery was dissected on the right side of the hilum and encircled with a vessel loop. Moreover, the right liver, including segment I, was mobilized from the retroperitoneum and from the vena cava. Finally, the right and middle hepatic veins were visualized; the middle hepatic vein was divided and the right hepatic vein was encircled with a vessel loop. Following placement of several drains, the abdomen was closed.

The patient recovered quickly from surgery; liver function was normal, and a computed tomography (CT) scan performed after 8 days (fig. 1b) astonishingly showed that the left lateral section had obviously increased to 723 ml, i.e. by more than 90%. Therefore, it was decided to perform completion surgery the following day. During this second operation, the distal bile duct, the right hepatic artery, and the right hepatic vein were divided, and the extended right liver including segment I was removed. Then, a systematic lymphadenectomy was performed prior to closure of the abdomen. The patient recovered quickly from surgery (fig. 1c) and could be discharged 10 days later.

Histology of the resected specimens showed a Klatskin tumor (hCCC) with 2 lymph node metastases as well as microscopic peritoneal carcinomatosis in the lesser omentum (pT3, pN1(2/8), $pM1_{per}$, local R0). As already suspected from this histology, the patient started to develop ascites and signs of overt peritoneal carcinomatosis about 6 months after surgery and died another 8 months later from tumor recurrence.

## Subsequent Patients Undergoing 'In-Situ Split' Liver Resection in Index Center

Although the technique had worked well and had led to very rapid hypertrophy of a rather small left lateral section, it was not applied again until more than half a year later (June 2008). At this time, it was used in a rather complex patient with rectal cancer and multiple synchronous liver metastases. After systemic chemotherapy, the first operation consisted of an abdominoperineal rectum resection with terminal descendostomy and 'in-situ splitting' of the liver. Liver segments II and III proved to be tumor-free on intraoperative ultrasound, while all other segments, including segment I, had tumor involvement. This time, the right portal vein was divided and the right hepatic artery marked with a vessel loop on the right side of the hilum, the right liver including segment I was mobilized from the vena cava, and the right hepatic vein was encircled with a vessel loop. Then the liver parenchyma was completely divided to the right of the falciform and round ligaments with the resection line then turning left in front of segment I. Finally, the middle hepatic vein was encircled with a vessel loop, and after placement of drains the operation was completed. Again, there was a rapid increase in the CT-measured volume of segments II and III from 211 ml prior to the first operation to 373 ml after 9 days (i.e. 76% volume increase) (fig. 2) so that the second surgery could be performed on day 10 with an uncomplicated postoperative course. Another patient, this time with metachronous colorectal liver metastases, underwent a similar procedure in September 2008. In this patient, an injury to the left bile duct occurred during the second surgery which was addressed by an end-to-end reconstruction of the duct. However, after a few days, biliary leakage required reoperation, which revealed necrosis of the duct at the anastomosis site so that a hepaticojejunostomy had to be performed. Again, after several days, leakage was noticed again with erosion bleeding from the hepatic artery, again necessitating emergency surgery. The patient finally died from multiorgan failure a few days later.

In 2009, the new technique was applied in 2 patients both suffering from intrahepatic cholangiocellular carcinoma (iCCC) (fig. 3a). In both patients, the 'standard' procedure was performed with complete parenchymal division to the right of the falciform and round ligaments, with a small part of subsegment IVa preserved in 1 of the 2 patients. These were the only 2 patients where the increase in volume of the left lateral section was below 50%, and in 1 patient the remnant liver volume prior to the second step of surgery even remained below 0.5% of the body weight; this patient had already undergone prior interventional embolization of the right portal vein without relevant hypertrophy of the left lateral section (fig. 3b). Nevertheless, the second step of surgery was performed (fig. 3c), and both patients recovered well.

In 2010, a total of 4 'in-situ split' liver resections were performed; 3 patients had colorectal metastases, and 1 patient suffered from metachronous liver metastases from cervical cancer.

In summary, all patients underwent extended right hepatectomy (trisectionectomy). Segment I had to be removed in about half of the patients and could be spared in the other half.

## Application of the Technique in Other Centers in Germany

Since the first case, the new technique was initially only informally communicated by the author and some of the senior surgeons of the department on a national level. It was then rapidly taken up and applied by a number of colleagues in Germany, particularly in Göttingen (Aiman Obed), Mainz (Hauke Lang), Tübingen (Silvio Nadalin and Alfred Königsrainer), Giessen (Winfried Padberg), and Hamburg (Karl Oldhafer). In order to accumulate an appropriate number of patients for the first report on this method, 5 German centers joined their experience with a total of

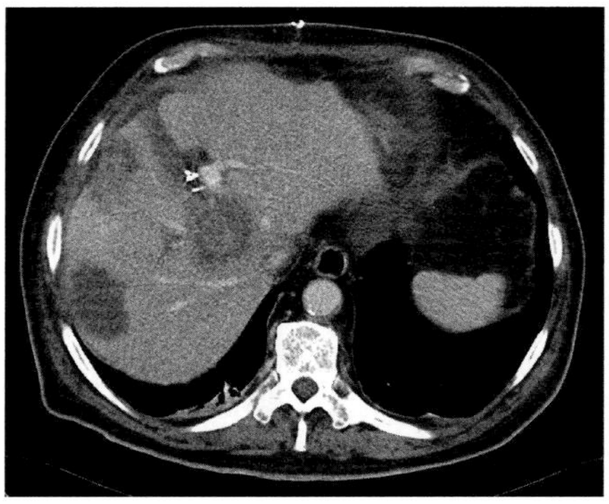

**Fig. 2.** Second patient undergoing 'in-situ split' liver resection/ALPPS in 2008, with rectal cancer and synchronous colorectal liver metastases. Contrast-enhanced computed tomography scan 8 days after the first surgery.

25 patients for analysis in 2011, which led to the sentinel publication of 'in-situ split' liver resection in *Annals of Surgery* in 2012 [5]. Since then, many German centers have embraced the new method.

## Application of the Technique Worldwide

The new technique appeared on the international podium when Hauke Lang presented 3 cases as a poster at the 9th E-AHPBA (European-African Hepato-Pancreato-Biliary Association) meeting in Cape Town, South Africa, in April 2011 [6], where it was viewed rather controversially. After this presentation, Eduardo de Santibañes from Buenos Aires was one of the first to pick up the idea and start using the concept outside of Europe. After the formal publication of the German cases in *Annals of Surgery* in March 2012 [5], the technique became known worldwide. An accompanying editorial of our paper by the journal editor Pierre-Alain Clavien together with Eduardo de Santibañes introduced the acronym 'ALPPS' for our 'in-situ split' liver resection [7]. In fact, the paper created enormous publicity for this method which then underwent various modifications by many groups worldwide, such as 'mini-ALPPS' [8], 'partial ALPPS' [9], and 'laparoscopic ALPPS' [10, 11]. In fact, more than 3,000 publications on this topic have appeared on PubMed since our initial description, and it has been the single focus of several conferences [12]. Moreover, an ALPPS registry was initiated, and already quite a number of publications have been generated from it and about 1,000 cases have been documented in it over the last 5 years [13, 14]. Most data in the registry come from centers in Europe (mainly Switzerland, Germany, France, Spain, UK, Belgium, Sweden) and from South America (Argentina, Brazil). Also, when looking at the published literature, it appears that the technique is now broadly used throughout the world, with the exception of the USA where only few surgeons seem to have embarked on it.

It is interesting that in some centers, 10–20% of all liver resection appear to be ALPPS resections. In our tertiary referral center, where about 200 mainly major liver resections are performed annually, we only come across about 4 cases per year where this approach is deemed helpful and necessary, representing about 2% of our caseload. In fact, in many cases of 'in-situ split'/ALPPS resection presented in reports and at conferences or documented in the

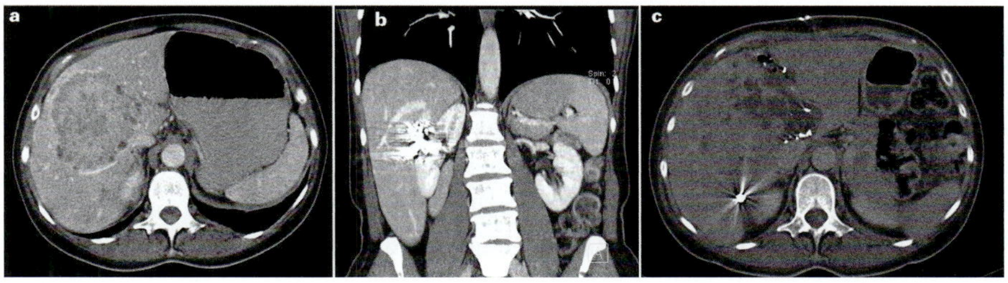

**Fig. 3.** Patient with intrahepatic cholangiocellular carcinoma (iCCC), after prior portal vein embolization (PVE), undergoing 'in-situ split' liver resection/ALPPS in 2009. **a** Contrast-enhanced computed tomography (CT) scan prior to the first surgery, post PVE; body weight 78 kg; left lateral section of the liver: 190 ml (0.24% of body weight). **b** Contrast-enhanced CT scan prior to first surgery, post PVE; embolization material in the right liver. **c** Contrast-enhanced CT scan prior to the second surgery after 9 days; body weight 78 kg; left lateral section: 275 ml (0.35% of body weight).

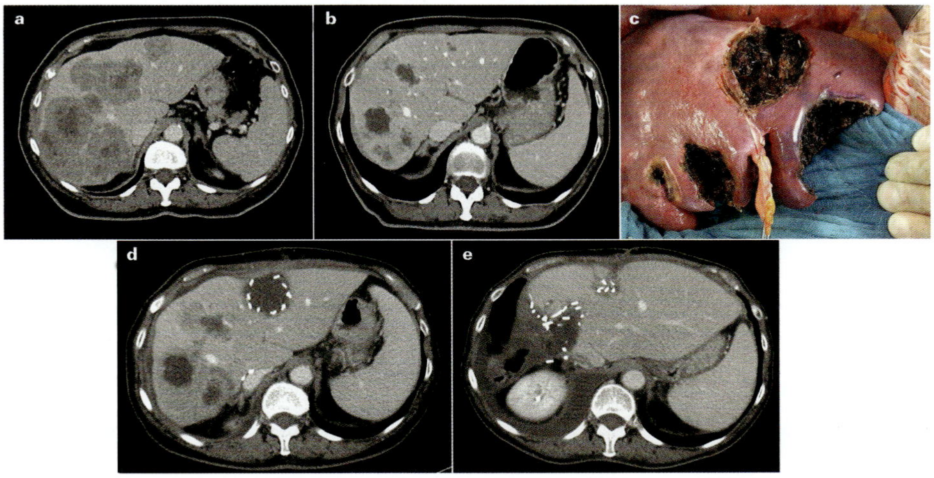

**Fig. 4.** Patient not suitable for 'in-situ split' liver resection/ALPPS but for 'standard' 2-stage hepatectomy (TSH), with synchronous colorectal liver metastases after neoadjuvant/conversion chemotherapy. **a** Contrast-enhanced computed tomography (CT) scan showing bilateral large colorectal liver metastases prior to chemotherapy. **b** Contrast-enhanced CT scan after 4 months of chemotherapy showing excellent response of the liver metastases, prior to the first surgery. **c** Intraoperative view at the end of the first surgery after resection of 5 metastases from the left (including segment IV) and the right portal vein division, in preparation for later removal of metastases on the right side by right hepatectomy. Preoperatively, 'in-situ split' liver resection/ALPPS had been planned; due to a larger than expected number of metastases in the left lobe (detected by intraoperative contrast-enhanced ultrasound), the strategy was changed intraoperatively. **d** Contrast-enhanced CT scan 8 weeks after primary surgery showing increase in volume of the left liver (including segments IV and I), prior to the second surgery following TSH/portal vein ligation. **e** Contrast-enhanced CT scan 5 weeks after the second surgery (right hepatectomy with minor parts of segment IVa).

registry, to our mind, this approach is neither necessary nor useful [13]. An example of such a patient with extensive colorectal liver metastases is demonstrated in figure 4.

## Discussion

The first case in which an 'in-situ split' liver resection was performed occurred spontaneously, i.e. without prior planning. The concept was developed intraoperatively to make an otherwise non-resectable tumor resectable, in a novel 2-stage procedure. This new procedure was based on extensive experience with complex liver resection and standard methods of parenchymal augmentation such as portal vein embolization (PVE) and 2-stage hepatectomy (TSH), as well as experience from the (mainly pediatric) field of split liver transplantation, namely 'in-situ splitting'. The approach was therefore termed 'in-situ split' liver resection. The spontaneous development of this technique demonstrates that in complex situations surgeons should try to find new solutions based on experiences even from a different surgical field. It also shows that new surgical strategies cannot always be designed by thoughtful planning and introduced systematically, but that spontaneous ideas can also be very fruitful.

Interestingly, the indication for the novel procedure in the first patient turned out to be rather suboptimal, and it has rarely been used for this indication since (including our center) [15–17]. However, a broad range of other indications in which the technique is useful have emerged and include many primary (predominantly hepatocellular carcinoma and iCCC) [18] as well as secondary liver tumors, i.e. metastases. In fact, as shown by the ALPPS registry data, colorectal liver metastases currently represent the primary indication for 'in-situ split' liver resection/ALPPS in our center and worldwide [14, 15, 19–22].

It has to be kept in mind that 'in-situ split' liver resection/ALPPS is not a completely novel technique standing on its own, but that it is rather an additional new tool in the surgical armament for the treatment of liver tumors. Compared to other available techniques, it has some advantages and some disadvantages, which have to be considered in the decision-making process in each individual case: i) interventional PVE (or surgical portal vein ligation) if hypertrophy of the complete left liver (including segment IV) is to be achieved; ii) TSH if volume increase is not specifically dependent on the left lateral section; iii) combination of resection and local ablation (either simultaneously or sequentially); and iv) 1-stage surgery, even when the volume of the remnant liver is marginally low. Thus, a comparison of the various techniques [22] is generally not very informative since all have slightly different indications. As mentioned above, in our tertiary referral center with about 200 (mostly major) liver resections per year, with the differential use of all the techniques, 'in-situ split' liver resection/ALPPS is performed in only about 2%, i.e. approximately 4 cases, per year.

Considering the literature on 'in-situ split' liver resection/ALPPS over the last 5 years, as well as listening to oral presentations about the topic, it emerges that many centers/surgeons use the technique for a much broader range of indications. These include cases of anatomic right hepatectomy as well as trisectionectomy in patients with an appropriately large remnant left lateral section, with or without segment I. It appears that many centers may use the method more frequently because it is currently 'fashionable', or because it is surgically and scientifically (publications) interesting, or in order to increase the competitiveness of the respective center (marketing). However, a highly sensible and selective use of the technique is essential in order to achieve the highest benefit and the lowest risk for each individual patient.

In conclusion, we are astonished at the publicity the 'in-situ split' liver resection/ALPPS procedure has gained; it has almost become a 'fashion'. We consider it less of a 'great new technique' but rather a new addition to the armament of highly experienced HPB surgeons. Every surgeon using this technique should have the entire spectrum of techniques and interventions available in order to select the optimal surgical approach for each individual patient. Sensible selection of patients who may benefit from the use of 'in-situ split' liver resection/ALPPS – with or without some of the modifications described in the recent literature or that may be developed in the future – is essential, as is the continued extensive (and truthful) discussion and reporting of results. Clearly no technique can overrule tumor biology [21].

## Disclosure Statement

There is no conflict of interest by any of the authors.

## References


1 Guglielmi A, Ruzzenente A, Conci S, Valdegamberi A, Iacono C: How much remnant is enough in liver resection? Dig Surg 2012;29:6–17.
2 Ironside N, Bell R, Bartlett A, McCall J, Powell J, Pandanaboyana S: Systematic review of perioperative and survival outcomes of liver resections with and without preoperative portal vein embolization for colorectal metastases. HPB (Oxford) 2017;19:559–566.
3 Pandanaboyana S, Bell R, Hidalgo E, Toogood G, Prasad KR, Bartlett A, Lodge JP: A systematic review and meta-analysis of portal vein ligation versus portal vein embolization for elective liver resection. Surgery 2015;157:690–698.
4 Shindoh J, Vauthey JN, Zimmitti G, Curley SA, Huang SY, Mahvash A, Gupta S, Wallace MJ, Aloia TA: Analysis of the efficacy of portal vein embolization for patients with extensive liver malignancy and very low future liver remnant volume, including a comparison with the associating liver partition with portal vein ligation for staged hepatectomy approach. J Am Coll Surg 2013;217:126–133.
5 Schnitzbauer AA, Lang SA, Goessmann H, Nadalin S, Baumgart J, Farkas SA, Fichtner-Feigl S, Lorf T, Goralcyk A, Hörbelt R, Kroemer A, Loss M, Rümmele P, Scherer MN, Padberg W, Königsrainer A, Lang H, Obed A, Schlitt HJ: Right portal vein ligation combined with in situ splitting induces rapid left lateral liver lobe hypertrophy enabling 2-staged extended right hepatic resection in small-for-size settings. Ann Surg 2012;255:405–414.
6 Baumgart J, Lang S, Lang H: A new method for induction of liver hypertrophy prior to right trisectionectomy: a report of three cases. HPB (Oxford) 2011;13: 71–72.
7 De Santibanes E, Clavien PA: Playing Play-doh to prevent postoperative liver failure: the 'ALPPS' approach. Ann Surg 2012;255:415–417.
8 De Santibanes E, Alvarez FA, Ardiles V, Pekolj J, de Santibanes M: Inverting the ALPPS paradigm by minimizing first stage impact: the mini-ALPPS technique. Langenbecks Arch Surg 2016;401:557–563.
9 Petrowsky H, Gyori G, de Oliveira M, Lesurtel M, Clavien PA: Is partial-ALPPS safer than ALPPS? A single-center experience. Ann Surg 2015;261:e90–92.
10 Machado MA, Makdissi FF, Surjan RC, Basseres T, Schadde E: Transition from open to laparoscopic ALPPS for patients with very small FLR: the initial experience. HPB (Oxford) 2017;19:59–66.
11 Edmondson MJ, Sodergren MH, Pucher PH, Darzi A, Li J, Petrowsky H, Campos RR, Serrablo A, Jiao LR: Variations and adaptations of associated liver partition and portal vein ligation for staged hepatectomy (ALPPS): many routes to the summit. Surgery 2016;159:1058–1072.
12 Oldhafer KJ, Stavrou GA, van Gulik TM; Core Group: ALPPS – where do we stand, where do we go?: eight recommendations from the first International Expert Meeting. Ann Surg 2016;263:839–841.
13 Schadde E, Ardiles V, Robles-Campos R, Malago M, Machado M, Hernandez-Alejandro R, Soubrane O, Schnitzbauer AA, Raptis D, Tschuor C, Petrowsky H, De Santibanes E, Clavien PA; ALPPS Registry Group: Early survival and safety of ALPPS: first report of the International ALPPS Registry. Ann Surg 2014;260: 829–836.
14 Schadde E, Schnitzbauer AA, Tschuor C, Raptis DA, Bechstein WO, Clavien PA: Systematic review and meta-analysis of feasibility, safety, and efficacy of a novel procedure: associating liver partition and portal vein ligation for staged hepatectomy. Ann Surg Oncol 2015;22:3109–3120.
15 Li J, Girotti P, Königsrainer I, Ladurner R, Königsrainer A, Nadalin S: ALPPS in right trisectionectomy: a safe procedure to avoid postoperative liver failure? J Gastrointest Surg 2013;17:956–961.
16 Lang H, de Santibanes E, Clavien PA: Outcome of ALPPS for perihilar cholangiocarcinoma: case-control analysis including the first series from the international ALPPS registry. HPB (Oxford) 2017;19:379–380.
17 Olthof PB, Coelen RJS, Wiggers JK, Groot Koerkamp B, Malago M, Hernandez-Alejandro R, Topp SA, Vivarelli M, Aldrighetti LA, Robles Campos R, Oldhafer KJ, Jarnagin WR, van Gulik TM: High mortality after ALPPS for perihilar cholangiocarcinoma: case-control analysis including the first series from the international ALPPS registry. HPB (Oxford) 2017;19: 381–387.
18 Vennarecci G, Grazi GL, Sperduti I, Busi Rizzi E, Felli E, Antonini M, D'Offizi G, Ettorre GM: ALPPS for primary and secondary liver tumors. Int J Surg 2016;30: 38–44.
19 Bjornsson B, Sparrelid E, Rosok B, Pomianowska E, Hasselgren K, Gasslander T, Bjornbeth BA, Isaksson B, Sandstrom P: Associating liver partition and portal vein ligation for staged hepatectomy in patients with colorectal liver metastases – intermediate oncological results. Eur J Surg Oncol 2016;42:531–537.
20 Lang SA, Loss M, Benseler V, Glockzin G, Schlitt HJ: Long-term results after in-situ split (ISS) liver resection. Langenbecks Arch Surg 2015;400:361–369.
21 Oldhafer KJ, Donati M, Jenner RM, Stang A, Stavrou GA: ALPPS for patients with colorectal liver metastases: effective liver hypertrophy, but early tumor recurrence. World J Surg 2014;38:1504–1509.
22 Ratti F, Schadde E, Masetti M, Massani M, Zanello M, Serenari M, Cipriani F, Bonariol L, Bassi N, Aldrighetti L, Jovine E: Strategies to increase the resectability of patients with colorectal liver metastases: a multi-center case-match analysis of ALPPS and conventional two-stage hepatectomy. Ann Surg Oncol 2015;22:1933–1942.

Visceral Medicine

Review Article

Visc Med 2017;33:414–417
DOI: 10.1159/000479474

Published online: November 22, 2017

# Portal Vein Embolization: History and Current Indications

Hiroji Shinkawa Shigekazu Takemura Shogo Tanaka Shoji Kubo

Department of Hepato-Biliary-Pancreatic Surgery, Osaka City University Graduate School of Medicine, Osaka, Japan

**Keywords**

Portal vein embolization · Hepatectomy · Future liver remnant

**Summary**

Portal vein embolization (PVE) was first adapted for patients undergoing major hepatectomy for hepatocellular carcinoma (HCC). In these patients, PVE caused hypertrophy of the unaffected liver and increased the volumetric ratio of future liver remnant (FLR) to total liver volume. $^{99m}$Technetium-galactosyl human serum albumin ($^{99m}$Tc-GSA) scintigraphy revealed that PVE also induced a shift in hepatic function from the embolized part to the nonembolized part of the liver. Various hepatobiliary malignancies can be treated using PVE, and PVE is increasingly being used to expand the indication for major hepatectomy in patients with initially insufficient FLR volume or function. The indication for PVE is determined by the underlying liver function and standardized FLR volume. In patients with chronic hepatitis, the histologic inflammatory activity was negatively correlated with the increase in FLR volume, and PVE is not suitable for patients with high serum 7s collagen concentrations (>8 ng/ml). This finding may predict the efficacy of PVE. PVE before major hepatectomy can act as a tolerance test to avoid postoperative hepatic failure. PVE also improved long-term survival after liver resection in patients with HCC. Presently, PVE is a safe and useful treatment for patients undergoing major hepatectomy.



## Introduction

In 1975, Honjo et al. [1] reported portal vein ligation (PVL) as a treatment for unresectable liver cancer. However, in their series, the effect of PVL was unclear because histologic examination of the affected cancer was not done. PVL requires laparotomy. Therefore, we developed the percutaneous transhepatic portal vein embolization (PVE) technique that does not require laparotomy, and investigated the anticancer effects of PVE on hepatocellular carcinoma (HCC). These results were first reported by Kinoshita et al. [2] of our group. PVE was first performed to strengthen the anticancer effects of transcatheter arterial embolization (TAE) in patients with HCC, followed by liver resection. We found that PVE was safer than TAE, and while strengthening the anticancer effects of TAE it also caused hypertrophy of the unaffected liver. We also performed experiments using rats to clarify that PVE caused hypertrophy of the unaffected liver and atrophy of the affected liver.

Since our first report [2], PVE has been increasingly used at various institutes to expand the indication for major hepatectomy in patients with initially insufficient future liver remnant (FLR) volume or function [3, 4]. The indication for PVE was also extended to various hepatobiliary malignancies, including HCC with portal thrombi, hilar carcinoma, and metastatic liver tumors [3, 4].

Here we introduce the clinical and experimental studies conducted by our group and the current indications for PVE.

## Development of Portal Vein Embolization

Several years before our first report [2], we performed percutaneous transhepatic portography to investigate the portal invasion of hepatobiliary malignancies and branching patterns of the portal vein in such patients. Conversely, TAE had been developed as a treatment for HCC. However, it was not effective for extracapsular invasion and portal thrombi at that time. Therefore, we attempted PVE during portography to strengthen the anticancer effects in patients with HCC. Under ultrasound guidance, we used a catheter introducer for the selective puncture of a portal branch and administered a fibrin mixture with added Lipiodol® (Guerbet, Villepinte, France) to the portal vein, using a balloon catheter to prevent scattering of the embolic materials. PVE was performed at the right portal vein, the left portal vein, and the more peripheral part of the intrahepatic portal vein in patients with HCC (fig. 1A–C). In patients with a large liver tumor compressing the first portal branches, transileocecal PVE was performed (fig. 1D). Immediately

KARGER

Fax +49 761 4 52 07 14
Information@Karger.com
www.karger.com



Accessible online at:
www.karger.com/vis

Shoji Kubo, MD, PhD
Department of Hepato-Biliary-Pancreatic Surgery
Osaka City University Graduate School of Medicine
1-4-3 Asahimachi, Abeno-ku, Osaka 545-8585, Japan
m7696493@msic.med.osaka-cu.ac.jp

after PVE, portal pressure increased from 20 to 140 cm $H_2O$. Most patients had abdominal discomfort or pain and fever after PVE. Serum aspartate aminotransferase (AST) and alanine aminotransferase (ALT) levels slightly increased and then decreased within 2 weeks after PVE. We also found that the indocyanine green retention rate at 15 min (ICGR15) slightly increased. On laparotomy, the appearance of the area affected by PVE varied depending on the state of embolization of the portal branch and recanalization of the occluded artery. The embolized area was dark red, which produced a demarcation line between the embolized and nonembolized parts of the liver. Regarding liver specimens, PVE caused necrosis of the extracapsular invasion, portal thrombi, and main tumor. In the noncancerous areas, we observed atrophy of the hepatic cells and dilatation of the sinusoids. In patients with portal thrombi, the portal thrombus was covered by embolic materials after PVE (fig. 2). We also found that the unaffected liver volume increased, especially when the right portal vein was embolized.

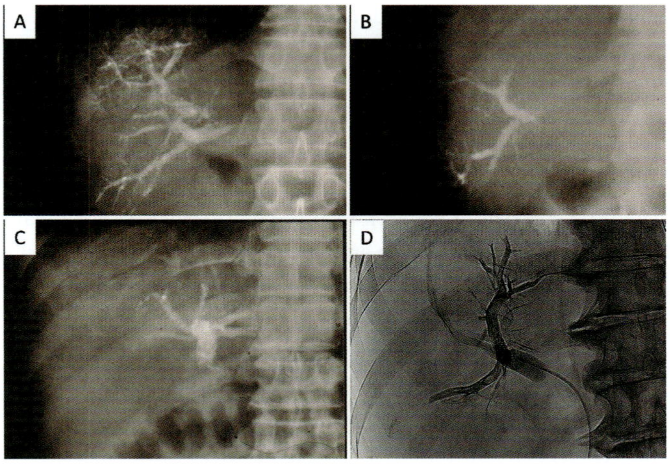


**Fig. 1.** Embolized portal veins: **A** right portal vein, **B** left portal vein, **C** posterior branch, and **D** transileocecal embolization of the right portal vein.

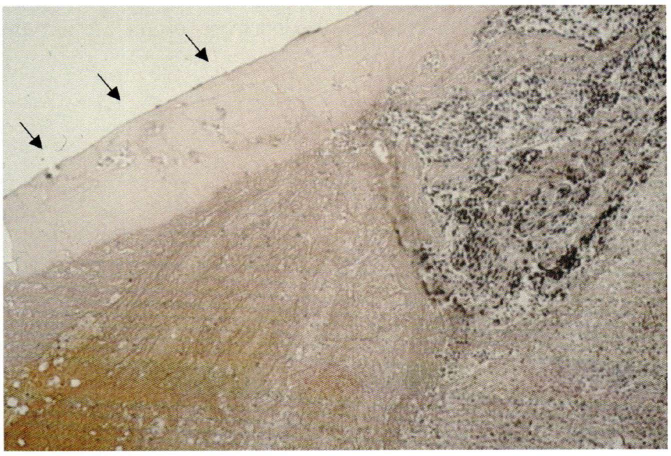

**Fig. 2.** Histologic finding after portal vein embolization in a patient with portal tumor thrombus. The tumor thrombus is covered by embolic material (arrows).

## Portal Vein Embolization before Major Hepatectomy

To determine whether PVE can extend surgical indications and increase the safety of liver resection, we studied the postoperative course of patients after major liver resection, i.e. right hepatectomy with and without PVE [5]. Serum AST, ALT, and total bilirubin levels and prothrombin time were not different between patients who did or did not undergo PVE. However, the pre- and postoperative changes in serum AST levels and prothrombin time were significantly smaller in patients who underwent PVE than in those who did not. In patients who underwent PVE, the left liver (nonembolized) volume increased after PVE and liver resection; however, when comparing the volume of the left liver at the beginning of treatment and 4 weeks after surgery, the extent of the volume increase in the left liver in patients who underwent PVE was similar to that in those who did not undergo PVE. This indicated that PVE causes regeneration of the left liver in two stages [6, 7].

$^{99m}$Technetium-galactosyl human serum albumin ($^{99m}$Tc-GSA) scintigraphy demonstrated that after PVE, the right receptor index decreased and the left receptor index increased (fig. 3) [8–10]. These results indicated that PVE induces a shift in hepatic function from the embolized to the nonembolized part of the liver, PVE of the right portal vein increases the hepatic functional reserve and left liver volume, and $^{99m}$Tc-GSA uptake after PVE may predict the response to liver resection. The status of liver regeneration after PVE can also be evaluated by the erythrocyte polyamine level [9].

The operative mortality after major hepatectomy was significantly lower in patients who underwent PVE than in those who did not. PVE also improved the outcomes after liver resection in patients with HCC [6, 7]. Previous reports have also demonstrated favorable long-term survival rates after PVE and subsequent major hepatectomy in patients with HCC, which were similar or superior to those in patients who did not undergo PVE [7, 10]. However, the recurrence-free survival rates were reportedly similar between patients who did and did not undergo PVE for HCC [7, 10, 11]. Beppu et al. [12] reported that even though patients with HCC who underwent preoperative PVE and right-sided hemihepatectomy had a significantly larger resected liver volume on admission, their long-term prognosis was comparable to that of patients who underwent upfront hepatectomy. They also reported that PVE might decrease extrahepatic recurrences.

Despite prior PVE, hepatic failure developed in some patients after major hepatectomy. In some, the portal pressure immediately after PVE was >30 cm $H_2O$ [13]. In others, the prognostic score [14] (calculated by age, parenchymal hepatic resection rate, and ICGR15) 2 weeks after PVE increased to >50 points. Thus, a portal pressure of >30 cm $H_2O$, i.e. portal hypertension, or a prognostic score of >50 points were significantly associated with postoperative hepatic failure [9]. This means that PVE can act as a tolerance test before major hepatectomy. In such patients with a risk of postoperative hepatic failure, the amount of liver to be resected should probably be limited, or another therapy should be attempted.

A study on the relationship between histologic inflammatory activity and increase in the left liver volume in patients with HCC and chronic hepatitis showed that histologic inflammatory activity was negatively correlated with increase in left liver volume, indicating that histologic inflammatory activity was the essential factor regulating liver regeneration after PVE in patients with chronic hepatitis [13].

To determine the limitations of PVE preoperatively, we investigated the correlation between serum type IV collagen 7s domain (7s collagen) concentrations and changes in the left liver volume after PVE [15]. The percent increase in the left liver volume negatively correlated with the pre-embolization serum 7s collagen concentration. In some patients with high serum 7s collagen concentrations (>8 ng/ml), the percent increase was <100% and right hepatectomy was not performed. The serum 7s collagen concentration correlated with the histologic activity score (activity of hepatitis) and the histologic fibrosis score (degree of hepatic fibrosis). These results indicate that serum 7s collagen concentration may predict the efficacy of PVE. PVE before right hepatectomy may not be indicated in patients with high serum 7s collagen concentrations because increases in the left liver volume are not expected in such patients.

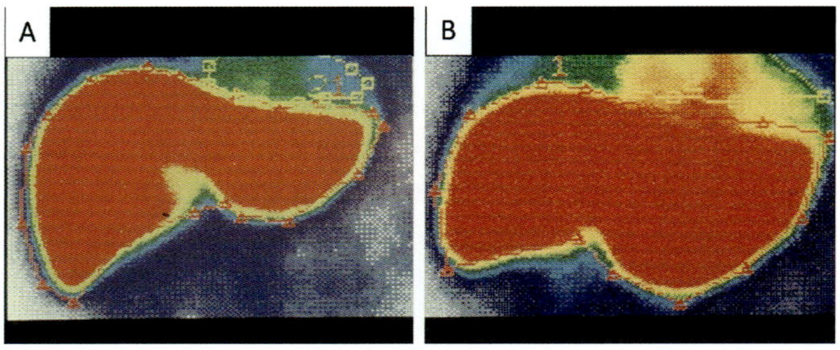


**Fig. 3.** $^{99m}$Technetium-galactosyl human serum albumin scintigraphy **A** before and **B** after right portal vein embolization.

## Experimental Study

For experimental study, we used rats in which the portal branches supplying 70% of the total liver volume were embolized (fig. 4) [16, 17]. Cirrhosis was induced by carbon tetrachloride because the background liver function in patients with HCC is frequently impaired by chronic liver disease such as cirrhosis. We showed that PVE caused an increase in ornithine decarboxylase activity, deoxyribonucleic acid (DNA) synthesis, and mitosis of the hepatocytes, although DNA synthesis was delayed in rats with cirrhosis. Thus, PVE caused cell proliferation and hypertrophy in the nonembolized part of the liver in normal rats and in those with cirrhosis.

We found that PVE enabled liver regeneration to occur in two stages, and prior PVE reduced the overload during the early stage of liver regeneration [17]. During the active phase of liver regeneration after hepatectomy, the basic functions of the hepatocytes such as albumin synthesis are depressed, indicating that the regenerating liver is vulnerable to stress. PVE of the right liver induced a shift in functional capacity from the right to the left liver without affecting total liver function so that when major hepatectomy is conducted, the basic functions of the left liver are already enhanced. PVE also enhanced the defense mechanisms of Kupffer cells. These mechanisms may contribute toward improving the outcome of major hepatectomy.

We then evaluated the effects of PVE in an endotoxin-induced liver injury model using rats. 7 days after PVE, the nonembolized part of the liver was approximately twice the size of the corresponding lobes in intact rats, the Kupffer cell density was doubled, and the hepatic function per unit weight, evaluated by the elimination of ICG, was approximately the same as that in the controls. When endotoxin was intravenously injected 48 h after hepatectomy in rats in whom previous PVE was and was not performed, hepatic dysfunction and endotoxin-induced liver injury were significantly less in the PVE + hepatectomy group than in the hepatectomy alone group. These results showed that preoperative PVE can make hepatectomy safer. However, drugs metabolized by cytochrome P450 (CYP) isoforms should be used carefully in patients who undergo major hepatectomy with PVE because the hepatic CYP-dependent drug metabolism by CYP isoforms recovered more slowly [18].

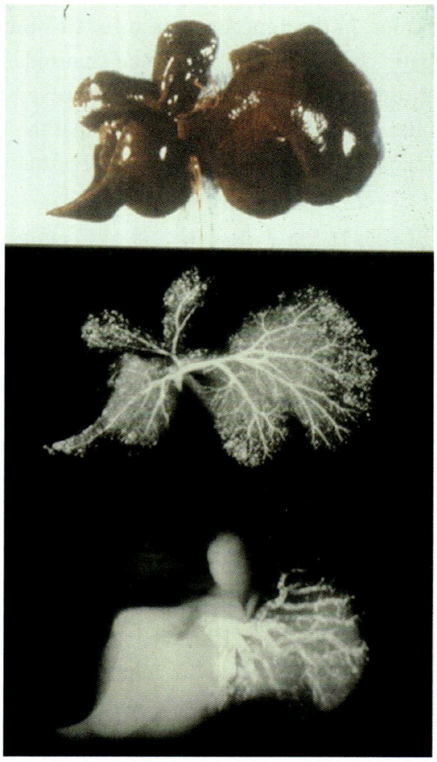

**Fig. 4.** The portal branches perfusing the median and left lateral lobes of the rat liver were embolized.

We also studied the effects of 70% PVL in rats. PVL caused increases in ornithine decarboxylase activity, DNA synthesis, and mitosis in the unaffected liver [19]. After PVL, a necrotic area appeared near the central vein, and it spread widely from the central to the intermediate zone of the hepatic lobules [20]. Subsequently, macrophages or Kupffer cells migrated to the extrasinusoidal space and the necrotic cells began to be eliminated by phagocytes. By day 14, the hepatic architecture had been completely restored. Some endothelial cells had lost their pore structures and had developed basement membranes. The Kupffer cell density and their phagocytic activity also decreased. Apoptotic hepatocytes were often seen. Therefore, the affected liver atrophied, although PVL caused regeneration of the unaffected liver.

## Current Indications of Portal Vein Embolization

In the current guidelines, PVE is indicated when the standardized FLR volume (percentage of total estimated liver volume) is ≤20% in a normal liver, ≤30% in liver with intermediate disease without cirrhosis, and ≤40% in liver with cirrhosis [21]. Patients classified as having Child-Pugh class B or C liver disease or those with ICGR15 > 20% are not candidates for major hepatectomy after PVE. Our previous study showed that the effects of PVE are not seen in patients with severe hepatic fibrosis (serum 7s collagen concentration, >8 ng/ml) and severe active hepatitis. When the portal pressure is >30 cm $H_2O$ after PVE, the amount of liver to be resected should probably be limited or another therapy should be attempted.

In patients with biliary obstruction due to tumor progression, biliary decompression before PVE was required to avoid injuring the dilated bile duct. PVE has recently been used before various types of surgeries. Nagino et al. [4] reported the usefulness of additional embolization of segment IV branches in right PVE in patients undergoing right trisectionectomy.

## Additional Indications of Portal Vein Embolization

Bile leakage, one of the most common complications after hepatic resection, is sometimes intractable. Use of PVE has been reported for the treatment of interrupted-type bile leakages to decrease bile production from the embolized part of the liver [22]. We also experienced a case of a patient with intractable bile leakage that was resolved by PVE [23]. In this case, the posterior branch of the bile duct was completely obstructed after anterior sectionectomy. Portal posterior branch embolization stopped the bile leakage. Thus PVE might be a nonsurgical option for the treatment of intractable bile leakage.

## Conclusion

Today PVE is used worldwide as a preoperative treatment to make major hepatectomy safer and to increase the number of patients undergoing hepatectomy.

## Disclosure Statement

The authors declare no conflict of interest. There is no funding to report.

## References

1 Honjo I, Suzuki T, Ozawa K, Takasan H, Kitamura O: Ligation of a branch of the portal vein for carcinoma of the liver. Am J Surg 1975;130:296–302.
2 Kinoshita H, Sakai K, Hirohashi K, Igawa S, Yamasaki O, Kubo S: Preoperative portal vein embolization for hepatocellular carcinoma. World J Surg 1986;10:803–808.
3 Makuuchi M, Thai BL, Takayasu K, Takayama T, Kosuge T, Gunven P, Yamazaki S, Hasegawa H, Ozaki H: Preoperative portal embolization to increase safety of major hepatectomy for hilar bile duct carcinoma: a preliminary report. Surgery 1990;107:521–527.
4 Nagino M, Kamiya J, Kanai M, Uesaka K, Sano T, Yamamoto H, Hayakawa N, Nimura Y: Right trisegment portal vein embolization for biliary tract carcinoma: technique and clinical utility. Surgery 2000;127:155–160.
5 Kubo S, Kinoshita H, Hirohashi K, Tanaka H, Tsukamoto T, Shuto T, Morimoto Y, Kanazawa A, Mikami S, Sakata C: Efficacy of preoperative portal vein embolization before major hepatectomy for patients with impaired liver function: a retrospective study. J Hepatobiliary Pancreat Surg 1997;4:365–372.
6 Fujio N, Sakai K, Kinoshita H, Hirohashi K, Kubo S, Iwasa R, Lee KC: Results of treatment of patients with hepatocellular carcinoma with severe cirrhosis of the liver. World J Surg 1989;13:211–217.
7 Tanaka H, Hirohashi K, Kubo S, Shuto T, Higaki I, Kinoshita H: Preoperative portal vein embolization improves prognosis after right hepatectomy for hepatocellular carcinoma in patients with impaired hepatic function. Br J Surg 2000;87:879–882.
8 Kubo S, Shiomi S, Tanaka H, Shuto T, Takemura S, Mikami S, Uenishi T, Nishino Y, Hirohashi K, Kawamura E, Kinoshita H: Evaluation of the effect of portal vein embolization on liver function by $^{99m}$Tc-galactosyl human serum albumin scintigraphy. J Surg Res 2002;107:113–118.
9 Tsukamoto T, Kinoshita H, Hirohashi K, Kubo S, Tanaka H, Otani S: Human erythrocyte polyamine levels after portal vein embolization. Hepatogastroenterology 1999;46:3178–3183.
10 Shindoh J, CW DT, Vauthey JN: Portal vein embolization for hepatocellular carcinoma. Liver Cancer 2012;1:159–167.
11 Kinoshita H, Hirohashi K, Kubo S: Preoperative portal vein embolization for hepatocellular carcinoma; in Tobe R, Kameda H, Okudaira M, Ohto M, Endo Y, Mito M, Okamoto E, Tanikawa K, Kojiro M (eds): Primary Liver Cancer in Japan. Tokyo, Springer, 1992, pp 283–290.
12 Beppu T, Okabe H, Okuda K, Eguchi S, Kitahara K, Taniai N, Ueno S, Shirabe K, Ohta M, Kondo K, Nanashima A, Noritomi T, Okamoto K, Kikuchi K, Baba H, Fujioka H: Portal vein embolization followed by right-side hemihepatectomy for hepatocellular carcinoma patients: a Japanese multi-institutional study. J Am Coll Surg 2016;222:1138–1148.
13 Tanaka H, Hirohashi K, Kubo S, Ikebe T, Tsukamoto T, Hamba H, Shuto T, Wakasa K, Kinoshita H: Influence of histological inflammatory activity on regenerative capacity of liver after percutaneous transhepatic portal vein embolization. J Gastroenterol 1999;34:100–104.
14 Okamoto E, Kyo A, Yamanaka N, Tanaka N, Kuwata K: Prediction of the safe limits of hepatectomy by combined volumetric and functional measurements in patients with impaired hepatic function. Surgery 1984;95:586–592.
15 Wu JS, Kubo S, Tanaka H, Shuto T, Takemura S, Tsukamoto T, Hirohashi K, Kinoshita H: Type IV collagen 7s domain as a predictor of poor efficacy of portal vein embolization before major hepatectomy. Surg Today 2005;35:41–46.
16 Lee KC, Kinoshita H, Hirohashi K, Kubo S, Iwasa R: Extension of surgical indications for hepatocellular carcinoma by portal vein embolization. World J Surg 1993;17:109–115.
17 Tanaka H, Kinoshita H, Hirohashi K, Kubo S, Lee KC: Increased safety by two-stage hepatectomy with preoperative portal vein embolization in rats. J Surg Res 1994;57:687–692.
18 Takemura S, Minamiyama Y, Hirohashi K, Kubo S, Funae Y, Kinoshita H: Recovery of hepatic function determined by cytochrome P450-dependent drug metabolism lags after compensatory hepatic volume changes after portal vein ligation in rats. J Surg Res 2006;134:285–291.
19 Kubo S, Matsui-Yuasa I, Otani S, Morisawa S, Kinoshita H, Sakai K: Effect of portal branch ligation on polyamine metabolism in rat liver. Life Sci 1986;38:1835–1840.
20 Tanaka H, Ikeda K, Matsuyama M, Kubo S, Hirohashi K, Kinoshita H: Morphological and functional changes after portal vein occlusion in rats. J Hepatobiliary Pancreat Surg 1997;4:365–372.
21 Vauthey JN, Dixon E, Abdalla EK, Helton WS, Pawlik TM, Taouli B, Brouquet A, Adams RB: Pretreatment assessment of hepatocellular carcinoma: expert consensus statement. HPB 2010;12:289–299.
22 Honore C, Vibert E, Hoti E, Azoulay D, Adam R, Castaing D: Management of excluded segmental bile duct leakage following liver resection. HPB 2009;11:364–369.
23 Hai S, Tanaka H, Takemura S, Sakabe K, Ichikawa T, Kubo S: Portal vein embolization for an intractable bile leakage after hepatectomy. Clin J Gastroenterol 2012;5:287–291.

Visceral Medicine

Review Article

Visc Med 2017;33:419–425
DOI: 10.1159/000480034

Published online: November 24, 2017

# Portal Vein Embolization: State-of-the-Art Technique and Options to Improve Liver Hypertrophy

Steven Y. Huang[a] Thomas A. Aloia[b]

[a]Department of Interventional Radiology, The University of Texas MD Anderson Cancer Center, Houston, TX, USA;
[b]Department of Surgical Oncology, The University of Texas MD Anderson Cancer Center, Houston, TX, USA

**Keywords**
PVE · Technique · Adjunctive options

**Summary**
Portal vein embolization (PVE) is associated with a high technical and clinical success rate for induction of future liver remnant hypertrophy prior to surgical resection. The degree of hypertrophy is variable and depends on multiple factors, including technical aspects of the procedure and underlying chronic liver disease. For patients with insufficient liver volume following PVE, adjunctive techniques, such as intra-portal administration of stem cells, dietary supplementation, transarterial embolization, and hepatic vein embolization, are available. Our purpose is to review the state-of-the-art technique associated with high-quality PVE and to discuss options to improve hypertrophy of the future liver remnant.



## Introduction

Postoperative liver insufficiency is a severe, life-threatening complication following surgical resection for primary and secondary liver cancer. The mortality following major liver resection ranges from 3.2 to 7% for patients with non-injured liver and up to 32% for patients with cirrhosis [1–3]. Most cases of mortality can be attributed to postoperative liver failure, which is related to the size and function of the liver remnant [4]. Preoperative portal vein embolization (PVE) increases the size of the future liver remnant (FLR) and is associated with an overall morbidity of 21.7% and an overall mortality of 3.3% following major liver resection [5]. PVE induces sufficient liver hypertrophy to allow 78–80% of patients to undergo major hepatectomy [6, 7]. The main causes of patient dropout following PVE are disease progression, medical comorbidities, and insufficient hypertrophy. The frequency of insufficient hypertrophy precluding definitive resection is only 0.6–3.6% [6, 7]. In these few cases, there are options to stimulate additional liver growth. Our purpose is to review the state-of-the-art technique associated with high-quality PVE and to discuss options to improve hypertrophy of the FLR.

## State-of-the-Art Technique for High-Quality Portal Vein Embolization

### *Planning*

Prior to performing PVE, multiple patient factors should be considered to optimize FLR growth. The degree of liver hypertrophy is affected by chronic liver disease [8, 9]. Thus, for some cases (e.g. patients with liver cirrhosis needing 40% FLR), optimal hypertrophy may require an adjunctive procedure, such as sequential transarterial embolization (TAE) and PVE to achieve sufficient hypertrophy (see chapter on 'Sequential TAE and PVE'). In addition to underlying liver disease, preoperative chemotherapy for patients with colorectal liver metastases induces agent-specific toxicities to the liver that affect patient outcomes [10]. While the effects of fluorouracil, oxaliplatin, and irinotecan on morbidity and mortality following major liver surgery have been reported [11–13], their impact on the efficacy of PVE to induce FLR hypertrophy is less certain. In 2006, Beal et al. [14] showed that oxaliplatin-based chemotherapy administered in the interval between PVE and resection impaired liver regeneration (p = 0.016). Additional recent studies by Goere et al. [15], Covey et al. [16], and Tanaka et al. [17] showed that chemotherapy did not impair liver hypertrophy. Thus, while surgeons may choose to withhold chemotherapy 4–6 weeks prior to resection to mitigate the risks posed by hepatotoxic chemotherapy to postoperative liver function, the published literature suggests that there is no significant effect upon liver regeneration following PVE.

KARGER

Fax +49 761 4 52 07 14
Information@Karger.com
www.karger.com



Accessible online at:
www.karger.com/vis

Steven Y. Huang, MD
Department of Interventional Radiology
The University of Texas MD Anderson Cancer Center
1515 Holcombe Blvd., Unit 1471, 77030 Houston, TX, USA
SYHuang@mdanderson.org

*Technique*

PVE can be performed with intravenous moderate sedation or general anesthesia. There is no consensus on the use of prophylactic antibiotics. If an antibiotic is administered, a single dose can be administered within 1 h of the procedure. A common choice is ceftriaxone (1 g intravenous) or vancomycin (15 mg/kg) if the patient is penicillin-allergic. Unlike TAE, there have been no reports of patients with prior biliary manipulation who develop an abscess following PVE.

PVE can be performed via a surgical transileocolic or percutaneous transhepatic approach. In a meta-analysis, Abulkhir et al. [18] found that the FLR hypertrophy was significantly higher using the transhepatic technique with no significant difference in major complications. Percutaneous ultrasound-guided transhepatic access into the portal system can be performed from the contralateral or ipsilateral side of the liver to be resected [19]. Advantages of contralateral liver access (i.e. access through the FLR) are i) ease of manipulating the catheter into the right liver lobe, ii) deployment of embolic material in the direction of portal blood flow, and iii) avoidance of puncturing tumors in the right hepatic lobe. Disadvantages include difficulty with maneuvering a catheter into the anterior branches of S4 and potential injury to the FLR. The technical challenge of embolization of the right portal vein branches from a peripheral right portal vein access can be mitigated with the use of reverse-curve catheters (e.g. SOS-2 Omni® Catheter, AngioDynamics, Queensbury, NY, USA). It should be noted that studies by Ribero et al. [20] and Di Stefano et al. [21] showed no difference in the type or rates of complications between contralateral or ipsilateral liver access.

The nuances of our technique for PVE at The University of Texas MD Anderson Cancer Center have been previously described [22]. In brief, access to a peripheral branch of the ipsilateral portal system can be obtained with ultrasound guidance. Following placement of a 6-French vascular sheath, an Omni™ flush catheter (AngioDynamics) is placed at the splenic vein-superior mesenteric vein confluence. Venogram is performed in the anterior-posterior, oblique, and craniocaudal projections to delineate the S4 portal veins as well as separate the anterior and posterior right portal vein branches. Measurement of portal pressures should be performed as this may influence the decision of whether to operate. Patients with portosystemic gradients >12 mm Hg are at major risk of perisurgical complications [23–25]. PVE should increase the portosystemic gradient by 3 mm Hg [23]. However, the effect of increased portal pressures following PVE on FLR hypertrophy, surgical outcomes, and evolution of portal hypertension is unclear.

PVE has been successfully performed with multiple agents either alone or in combination: particulates (i.e., polyvinyl alcohol (PVA) or trisacryl gelatin microspheres), n-butyl cyanoacrylate (NBCA), absorbable gelatin, ethanol, fibrin glue, and sclerosants (e.g. Aethoxysclerol/air-foam) [5]. Embolization should be permanent and as far distal as possible. Proximal embolization with coils without more distal particulate or liquid embolization allows intraparenchymal shunts to develop and limits FLR hypertrophy [22]. Of the various embolic agents, absorbable gelatin is associated with portal venous recanalization as early as 2 weeks following embolization [19, 26]. In a report of 44 patients, Madoff et al. [27] found larger FLR hypertrophy following right portal vein embolization (RPVE) extended to segment 4 (RPVE+4) with trisacryl microspheres (100–700 μm) when compared with PVA particles (355–1,000 μm). The two most commonly used agents used for portal venous occlusion are i) trisacryl microspheres with coil occlusion of the proximal right portal vein trunk and ii) NBCA (Histoacryl®, B Braun, Melsungen, Germany) mixed with ethiodized oil (Lipiodol®, Guerbet, Roissy, France). When performing particulate embolization with trisacryl microspheres, most surgeons will start with 100–300 μm particles, increasing in a stepwise fashion to 500–700 μm particles as hepatopedal flow is reduced. Coils are then placed at the origin of the segmental portal veins. Coil or vascular plug occlusion of the main right portal vein is an acceptable alternative to segmental venous coil occlusion so long as the operator can preserve at least 1 cm of patent right portal vein to facilitate surgical ligation. NBCA embolization involves injection of small aliquots of NBCA mixed with ethiodized oil in ratios of 1:2–1:8 with copious intermittent flushing using a nonionic solution such as 5% dextrose to prevent premature NBCA polymerization [22, 28]. In practice, a 1–3 ml syringe containing the NBCA mixed with ethiodized oil is connected to a 3-way stopcock in addition to a 20 ml syringe containing 5% dextrose. The main advantages of NBCA embolization are shorter procedure times, permanent aggressive distal embolization, and lower cost. It should be noted that NBCA induces a strong inflammatory response which can make resection more technically challenging [19]. Many embolic agents have been used to successfully increase the size of the FLR. Operator familiarity and experience with the embolic agent is of utmost importance to ensure precise delivery and preservation of non-targeted branches.

RPVE should be readily extended to segment 4 portal veins (RPVE+4) to enhance the degree of hypertrophy for segments 2 and 3. In a study of 73 patients who underwent RPVE (n = 15) or RPVE+4 (n = 58), volumes of segments 2 and 3 increased more in the RPVE+4 group (mean 141 ml for RPVE+4 compared to 106 ml for RPVE alone; p = 0.044). No significant differences between complication rates were identified [29]. Prior to embolization of segment 4, dedicated left portal venogram should be performed to delineate anatomy and patency. From an ipsilateral approach, segment 4 embolization is performed prior to RPVE as manipulating a catheter through an embolized right liver could cause dislodgement of embolic particles. Catheterization of segment 4 is performed with a Cobra-2 catheter (AngioDynamics). To prevent reflux of particles into the FLR, distal embolization is performed through a microcatheter. Alternatively, a balloon occlusion catheter can also be used to prevent reflux into the FLR (fig. 1). Coil embolization is then performed with pushable or detachable 0.018" microcoils (VortX, Interlock-18, Boston Scientific, Malborough, MA, USA). Operators who perform RPVE with NBCA mixed with ethiodized oil will often use particles and coils to embolize S4 branches because of the increased control offered by these agents.

The embolization endpoint for PVE should be complete stasis.

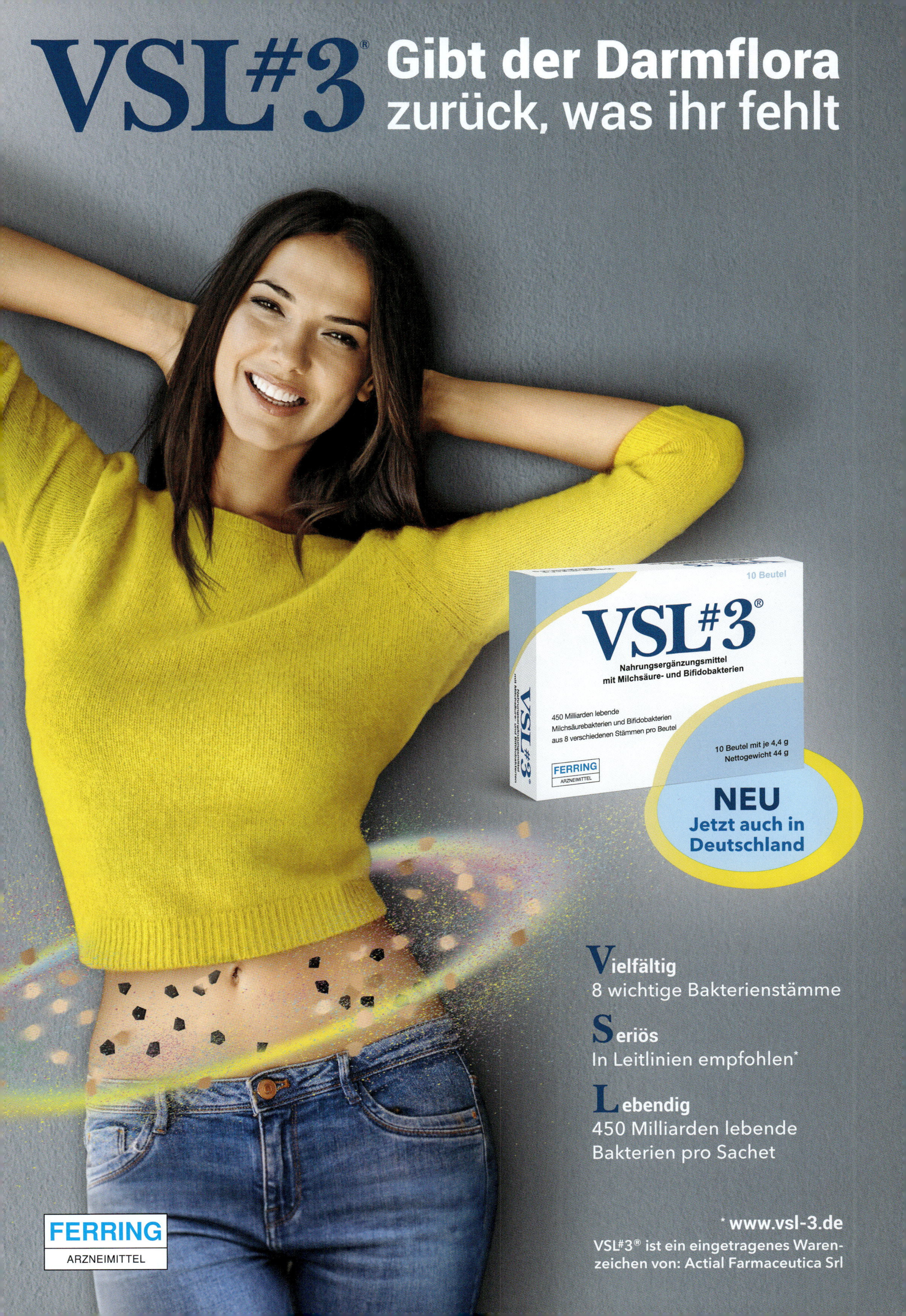

VSL#3® Gibt der Darmflora zurück, was ihr fehlt
10 Beutel
VSL#3®
Nahrungsergänzungsmittel mit Milchsäure- und Bifidobakterien
450 Milliarden lebende Milchsäurebakterien und Bifidobakterien aus 8 verschiedenen Stämmen pro Beutel
10 Beutel mit je 4,4 g Nettogewicht 44 g
FERRING ARZNEIMITTEL
NEU
Jetzt auch in Deutschland
Vielfältig
8 wichtige Bakterienstämme
Seriös
In Leitlinien empfohlen*
Lebendig
450 Milliarden lebende Bakterien pro Sachet
FERRING
ARZNEIMITTEL
* www.vsl-3.de
VSL#3® ist ein eingetragenes Warenzeichen von: Actial Farmaceutica Srl

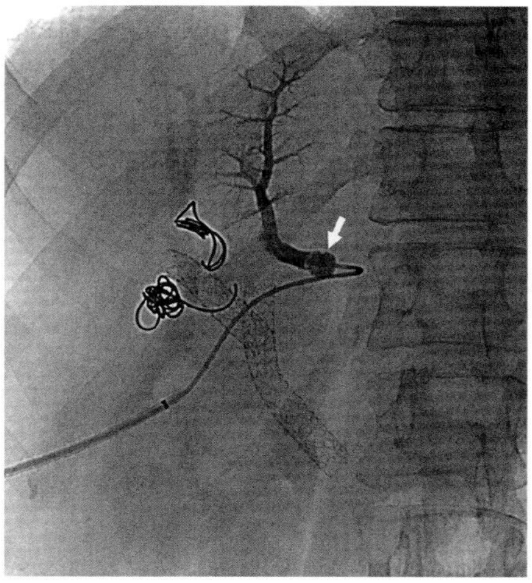


**Fig. 1.** 60-year-old female with cholangiocarcinoma presenting for right portal vein embolization extended to segment 4 portal veins. A balloon occlusion catheter (Fogarty®, Edwards Lifesciences, Irvine, CA, USA) is placed in segment 4A (white arrow). Injection of contrast demonstrates patent antegrade flow and no reflux. Image courtesy of Armeen Mahvash, MD.

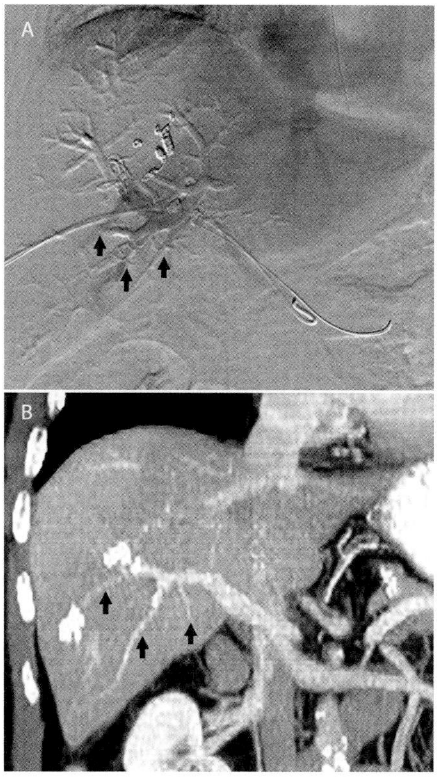


**Fig. 2.** 59-year-old male with metastatic colorectal carcinoma presenting for right portal vein embolization extended to segment 4 portal veins (RPVE+4) prior to extended right hepatectomy. **A** Completion portal venogram following embolization demonstrates sluggish but patent flow in 3 branches supplying segment 6 (black arrows). **B** Coronal maximum intensity projection image from a computed tomography scan performed 30 days following RPVE+4 demonstrates patent flow involving 3 branches supplying segment 6 (black arrows).

Termination of embolization prior to this endpoint incurs the risk of incomplete embolization and vessel recanalization, which limits hypertrophy (fig. 2). Assessment of stasis can be performed with portal venography. Theoretically, performing a post embolization venogram from an ipsilateral access requires manipulation of a catheter through the embolized lobe. In our practice, we generally advance the reverse-curve catheter used for particulate and coil embolization of the right portal vein into the main portal vein without changing to a multi-sidehole catheter. This allows for completion venography and measurement of post-embolization portal pressures while mitigating the risk associated with catheter manipulation and exchange.

*Complications*

In a large review of 1,179 patients who underwent PVE, van Lienden et al. [5] calculated a procedural-related mortality of 0.1% and a major complication rate of 0.4%. Major complications included vascular injury, biloma, infection, non-target embolization, portal/mesenteric venous thrombosis, and portal hypertension. Minor complications were generally self-limited and included fever (36.9%), elevation of transaminases (34.8%), abdominal discomfort/pain (22.9%), nausea/vomiting (2.0%), and ileus (1.2%).

## Options to Improve Future Liver Remnant Hypertrophy

*Intra-Portal Administration of Stem Cells*

To improve FLR hypertrophy following PVE, Schulte am Esch et al. [30] performed a study on 22 patients comparing PVE in combination with simultaneous administration of CD133+ bone marrow stem cells versus PVE alone. The authors found an absolute gain of 138.66 ± 66.29 ml in the PVE and stem cell group compared with 62.95 ± 40.03 ml in the PVE alone group ($p = 0.004$). These results corroborated an earlier pilot study conducted by Fürst et al. [31] in which the relative gain in FLR volume for patients administered stem cells following PVE (n = 6) was 77.3 ± 38.2% compared with 39.1 ± 20.4% for patients following PVE alone (n = 7) ($p = 0.039$). While the data is encouraging, several issues should be investigated prior to widespread adoption. The efficacy of this technique in patients with diabetes mellitus, chronic liver disease, and prolonged chemotherapy is unknown. There is also the possibility that administration of bone marrow stem cells may enhance tumor progression [32].

*Dietary Supplementation*

Dietary supplementation to improve the hypertrophic effect of PVE is an area of active research. In a preclinical study using New Zealand White rabbits, Olthof et al. [33] found that administration of obeticholic acid (OCA, potent farnesoid X receptor agonist) in addition to PVE resulted in FLR hypertrophy of 56.1 ± 20.3% compared to 26.1 ± 15.4% for control animals who underwent PVE only ($p < 0.001$). The number of Ki-67-positive hepatocytes was 1.6-fold higher in the animals administered OCA ($p = 0.045$), indicating a stronger hyperplastic hepatocyte response. Beppu et al. [34] conducted a small randomized clinical study in which one cohort (n = 13) was administered branched-chain amino acid dietary supplements (LIVACT®, Ajinomoto, Tokyo, Japan) before PVE and continued for 6 months following liver resection compared to another cohort (n = 15) who underwent PVE without dietary supplementation. Functional liver regeneration was assessed by liver uptake on Technetium-99m (Tc-99m) galactosyl human serum albumin scintigraphy. The authors found that the liver uptake value increased 266.7% in the branched-chain amino acid + PVE group compared to 77.6% for the PVE alone group ($p = 0.04$). While ad-

**Table 1.** Studies evaluating the effect of sequential transarterial chemoembolization (TACE) followed by portal vein embolization (PVE)

| Study [ref.] | n | Tumor | TACE technique | Time interval between TACE and PVE, weeks | FLR hypertrophy, % | Complications following TACE/PVE |
|---|---|---|---|---|---|---|
| Yamakado et al. [51] | 7 | HCC | TACE with ethiodized oil | 2–6 | 56.7 ± 21.6[a] | NA |
| Aoki et al. [36] | 17 | HCC | TACE with ethiodized oil | 1–1.5 | 51 (39–68)[b] | 5[c] |
| Ogata et al. [35] | 18 | HCC | TACE with ethiodized oil | 3–6 | 12 ± 5[a] | none |
| Peng et al. [52] | 29 | multiple | i) TACE with ethiodized oil<br>ii) drug-eluting beads | 8.6 (4–14.6)[b] | 7.4 (2.2–11.6)[b] | 1[d] |

[a]Mean ± standard deviation.
[b]Median (range).
[c]Included cholecystitis, pleural effusion, asthma attack, ascites, and bowel obstruction.
[d]Included abscess following arterial embolization.
FLR = Future liver remnant; HCC = hepatocellular carcinoma; NA = not applicable.

ditional research is needed, dietary supplementation is an intriguing field which may improve the hypertrophic and functional response of the FLR following PVE.

*Sequential TAE and PVE*

PVE reproducibly increases the size of the FLR though the degree of hypertrophy is variable, especially in patients with chronic liver disease [3]. Furthermore, for patients with hepatocellular carcinoma (HCC) and liver cirrhosis, arterioportal shunts in tumors may attenuate the hypertrophic effect of PVE. It has been shown that sequential TAE followed by PVE increases the rate of FLR hypertrophy more than PVE alone (table 1). The benefits of this dual technique are improved FLR hypertrophy relative to PVE alone and induction of an anti-tumor effect in the embolized lobe [35, 36]. For safety purposes, tumor embolization should be performed as far distally as possible, and liver functional tests should be allowed to normalize prior to PVE. Despite this cautious approach, Aoki et al. [36] demonstrated areas of segmental infarction within noncancerous liver of resected liver specimens. While embolization of the hepatic artery prior to PVE is an effective adjunctive technique, it should be performed carefully, since many of these patients have pre-existing liver dysfunction.

*Sequential PVE and TAE*

Definitive hepatectomy following PVE may not be possible because of disease progression, medical comorbidities, and insufficient hypertrophy of the FLR. For patients with HCC, TAE may be the next therapeutic option. A prior report by Kang et al. [37] showed that PVE followed by subselective TAE is a safe and effective technique to treat HCC. In addition to locoregional management of liver cancer, several small studies postulate that subsequent arterial embolization following PVE may further augment FLR hypertrophy [38–41]. Inaba et al. [39] found a change in FLR of 1.4 times that of the original level for combined PVE followed by TAE (n = 4 patients) compared to a change in FLR of 1.3 times that of the original level for the PVE-only group (n = 6). As expected, sequential PVE followed by TAE is associated with hepatic infarction and abscess formation [37, 38, 41]. To mitigate these risks, operators need to consider the type of embolic material, territory of embolization, and embolization endpoint carefully. The data currently available do not support any particular regimen. It is imperative that patients who undergo this sequential procedure be carefully selected and monitored following embolization.

*Sequential PVE and Hepatic Vein Embolization*

Hepatic vein embolization (HVE) following PVE induces further damage to the embolized lobe by increasing outflow obstruction, which obstructs arterial inflow and further decreases any residual portal blood flow. Hwang et al. [42] demonstrated the initial safety and efficacy of this technique in 12 patients with hepatobiliary malignancy. Because of insufficient FLR hypertrophy following RPVE, patients underwent right HVE (fig. 3). A vascular plug was placed at the central portion of the right hepatic vein, and all sizeable branches were embolized with coils. In a subsequent study, Hwang et al. [43] treated 42 patients over an 8-year period with insufficient FLR hypertrophy following PVE with adjunctive HVE. 33 (78.6%) of the patients had cholangiocarcinoma. The degree of FRL hypertrophy for this cohort was 13.3% following PVE and 28.9% following PVE-HVE. There were no procedural-related complications. As expected, histologic examination of the liver from resected specimens showed increased apoptosis in areas affected by both PVE and HVE compared to areas affected by PVE alone [42, 43]. Though the current clinical experience is limited, HVE following PVE appears to be effective and well-tolerated by patients with insufficient FLR hypertrophy following PVE.

*Simultaneous PVE and HVE (Liver Venous Deprivation)*

Liver venous deprivation (LVD) builds upon the earlier work by Hwang et al. [43]. The technique involves RPVE and embolization of the right and/or middle hepatic vein during the same procedure. An initial pilot study involving 7 patients by Guiu et al. [44] reported an FLR increase from 28.2% (range 22.4–33.3%) to 40.9% (range 33.6–59.3%) at 23 days following LVD. In a follow-up study of 10 patients, FLR volume increased by 53.4% as early as 7 days following LVD. Liver function as measured by Tc-99m mebrofenin hepatobiliary scintigraphy increased by 64.3% (range 28.1–107.5%)

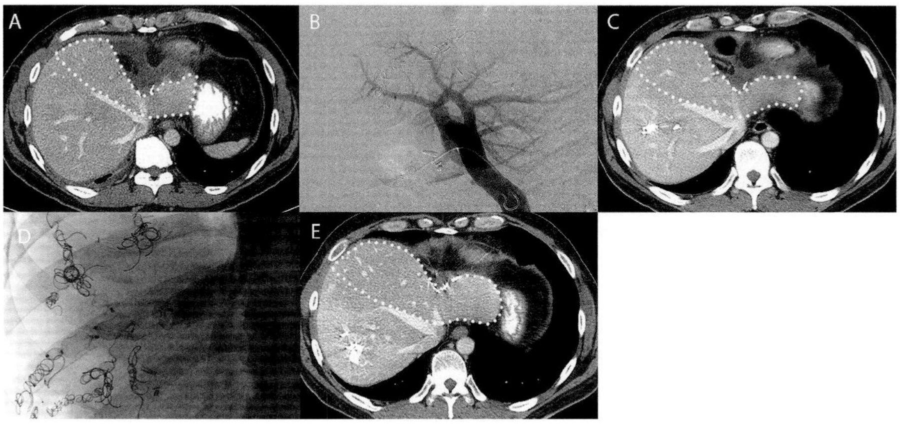


**Fig. 3.** 50-year-old male with metastatic colon cancer to the liver status post 1st-stage segment 3 liver resection presenting for right portal vein embolization (RPVE) prior to 2nd-stage right hepatectomy. **A** Axial computed tomography (CT) image demonstrates the future liver remnant (FLR, outlined by white dots) measuring 511 ml. **B** Patient underwent RPVE with trisacryl gelatin microspheres and coils. Completion portal venogram demonstrates successful occlusion of the right portal vein branches. **C** Axial CT image obtained 21 days following PVE demonstrates slight increase in FLR volume to 579 ml. **D** Patient underwent adjunctive right hepatic vein embolization (HVE) with coils and vascular plugs. Completion venogram demonstrates occlusion of the right hepatic vein. **E** Axial CT image from a CT scan obtained 57 days following HVE demonstrates interval increase in FLR volume to 740 ml.

at day 21. The procedure was relatively well-tolerated. Patients complained of fatigue (n = 2), fever (n = 3), and pain for 24 h (n = 6). Histology in the embolized lobe revealed sinusoidal dilatation, hepatocyte necrosis, and atrophy [45]. In another small study involving 7 patients, Le Roy et al. [46] found a mean FLR hypertrophy rate of 52.6% (range 18.2–187.9%) following LVD. There were no postprocedural complications. To date, there have been 17 published patients who have undergone LVD, and 3 (17.6%) patients did not undergo surgical resection. 2 patients experienced interval disease progression, and 1 patient had insufficient FLR hypertrophy. No patients who underwent surgery developed postoperative liver failure [44–46]. While these early results with LVD are encouraging, comparison studies are necessary to evaluate the additional benefit provided by simultaneous PVE and HVE.

*Sequential PVE and Parenchymal Liver Transection ('Salvage' ALPPS)*

'Salvage' ALPPS (associating liver partition and portal vein ligation for staged hepatectomy) involves parenchymal transection along the FLR margin. This procedure has been reported for patients with insufficient FLR hypertrophy following PVE [47–49]. Mean FLR hypertrophy after sequential PVE and ALPPS ranges from 57 to 65% [48, 49]. A recent consensus statement from an international expert meeting on ALPPS recommended that adjunctive ALPPS can be considered for patients with insufficient hypertrophy following PVE.

There are no prospective randomized clinical studies to prove the efficacy of PVE to prevent post-resection liver insufficiency or failure. As a result, physicians' knowledge and attitudes towards PVE are formed largely from retrospective data and personal experience. In a multinational study involving 54 institutions, Day et al. [50] found significant variability in surgeons' utilization of and attitudes towards PVE for FLR hypertrophy. Institutions capable of performing high-quality PVE (i.e. RPVE+4 and embolization with a permanent embolic agent such as trisacryl microspheres) were significantly associated with the subjective impression of a higher likelihood of FLR hypertrophy. The authors postulate that institutions without access to high-quality PVE are more likely to turn to the ALPPS procedure. Thus, it is important that for each case of insufficient FLR hypertrophy, the technique and materials used during PVE should be re-evaluated to assess whether liver growth was suboptimal because of technique or an intrinsic problem of liver regeneration. Research focused on patient selection will help to ensure that patients are provided upfront with the safest and most effective modality to maximize FLR hypertrophy.

## Conclusion

PVE has improved the safety profile for patients who undergo partial hepatectomy for more than 20 years. The technical and clinical success rate of PVE for the induction of FLR hypertrophy is high [6, 7]. Nonetheless, the degree of hypertrophy among patients is variable and may depend on multiple factors, including technical aspects of the procedure and underlying chronic liver disease. Adjunctive techniques to further improve FLR hypertrophy are becoming more prevalent. These interventions will continue to improve patient safety while eliminating cases of insufficient liver hypertrophy.

## Disclosure Statement

The authors S.Y.H. and T.A.A. report no conflict of interests.

## References


1 Broering DC, Hillert C, Krupski G, Fischer L, Mueller L, Achilles EG, Schulte am Esch J, Rogiers X: Portal vein embolization vs. portal vein ligation for induction of hypertrophy of the future liver remnant. J Gastrointest Surg 2002;6:905–913; discussion 913.

2 Hemming AW, Reed AI, Howard RJ, Fujita S, Hochwald SN, Caridi JG, Hawkins IF, Vauthey JN: Preoperative portal vein embolization for extended hepatectomy. Ann Surg 2003;237:686–691; discussion 691–693.

3 Farges O, Belghiti J, Kianmanesh R, Regimbeau JM, Santoro R, Vilgrain V, Denys A, Sauvanet A: Portal vein embolization before right hepatectomy: prospective clinical trial. Ann Surg 2003;237:208–217.

4 Yamanaka N, Okamoto E, Kuwata K, Tanaka N: A multiple regression equation for prediction of posthepatectomy liver failure. Ann Surg 1984;200:658–663.

5 Van Lienden KP, van den Esschert JW, de Graaf W, Bipat S, Lameris JS, van Gulik TM, van Delden OM: Portal vein embolization before liver resection: a systematic review. Cardiovasc Intervent Radiol 2013;36:25–34.

6 Yamashita S, Sakamoto Y, Yamamoto S, Takemura N, Omichi K, Shinkawa H, Mori K, Kaneko J, Akamatsu N, Arita J, Hasegawa K, Kokudo N: Efficacy of preoperative portal vein embolization among patients with hepatocellular carcinoma, biliary tract cancer, and colorectal liver metastases: a comparative study based on single-center experience of 319 cases. Ann Surg Oncol 2017;24:1557–1568.

7 Shindoh J, Tzeng CW, Aloia TA, Curley SA, Huang SY, Mahvash A, Gupta S, Wallace MJ, Vauthey JN: Safety and efficacy of portal vein embolization before planned major or extended hepatectomy: an institutional experience of 358 patients. J Gastrointest Surg 2014;18:45–51.

8 Azoulay D, Castaing D, Krissat J, Smail A, Hargreaves GM, Lemoine A, Emile JF, Bismuth H: Percutaneous portal vein embolization increases the feasibility and safety of major liver resection for hepatocellular carcinoma in injured liver. Ann Surg 2000;232:665–672.

9 Tanaka H, Hirohashi K, Kubo S, Shuto T, Higaki I, Kinoshita H: Preoperative portal vein embolization improves prognosis after right hepatectomy for hepatocellular carcinoma in patients with impaired hepatic function. Br J Surg 2000;87:879–882.

10 Zorzi D, Laurent A, Pawlik TM, Lauwers GY, Vauthey JN, Abdalla EK: Chemotherapy-associated hepatotoxicity and surgery for colorectal liver metastases. Br J Surg 2007;94:274–286.

11 Vauthey JN, Pawlik TM, Ribero D, Wu TT, Zorzi D, Hoff PM, Xiong HQ, Eng C, Lauwers GY, Mino-Kenudson M, Risio M, Muratore A, Capussotti L, Curley SA, Abdalla EK: Chemotherapy regimen predicts steatohepatitis and an increase in 90-day mortality after surgery for hepatic colorectal metastases. J Clin Oncol 2006;24:2065–2072.

12 Karoui M, Penna C, Amin-Hashem M, Mitry E, Benoist S, Franc B, Rougier P, Nordlinger B: Influence of preoperative chemotherapy on the risk of major hepatectomy for colorectal liver metastases. Ann Surg 2006;243:1–7.

13 Nakano H, Oussoultzoglou E, Rosso E, Casnedi S, Chenard-Neu MP, Dufour P, Bachellier P, Jaeck D: Sinusoidal injury increases morbidity after major hepatectomy in patients with colorectal liver metastases receiving preoperative chemotherapy. Ann Surg 2008;247:118–124.

14 Beal IK, Anthony S, Papadopoulou A, Hutchins R, Fusai G, Begent R, Davies N, Tibballs J, Davidson B: Portal vein embolisation prior to hepatic resection for colorectal liver metastases and the effects of periprocedure chemotherapy. Br J Radiol 2006;79:473–478.

15 Goere D, Farges O, Leporrier J, Sauvanet A, Vilgrain V, Belghiti J: Chemotherapy does not impair hypertrophy of the left liver after right portal vein obstruction. J Gastrointest Surg 2006;10:365–370.

16 Covey AM, Brown KT, Jarnagin WR, Brody LA, Schwartz L, Tuorto S, Sofocleous CT, D'Angelica M, Getrajdman GI, DeMatteo R, Kemeny NE, Fong Y: Combined portal vein embolization and neoadjuvant chemotherapy as a treatment strategy for resectable hepatic colorectal metastases. Ann Surg 2008;247:451–455.

17 Tanaka K, Kumamoto T, Matsuyama R, Takeda K, Nagano Y, Endo I: Influence of chemotherapy on liver regeneration induced by portal vein embolization or first hepatectomy of a staged procedure for colorectal liver metastases. J Gastrointest Surg 2010;14:359–368.

18 Abulkhir A, Limongelli P, Healey AJ, Damrah O, Tait P, Jackson J, Habib N, Jiao LR: Preoperative portal vein embolization for major liver resection: a meta-analysis. Ann Surg 2008;247:49–57.

19 De Baere T, Roche A, Elias D, Lasser P, Lagrange C, Bousson V: Preoperative portal vein embolization for extension of hepatectomy indications. Hepatology 1996;24:1386–1391.

20 Ribero D, Abdalla EK, Madoff DC, Donadon M, Loyer EM, Vauthey JN: Portal vein embolization before major hepatectomy and its effects on regeneration, resectability and outcome. Br J Surg 2007;94:1386–1394.

21 Di Stefano DR, de Baere T, Denys A, Hakime A, Gorin G, Gillet M, Saric J, Trillaud H, Petit P, Bartoli JM, Elias D, Delpero JR: Preoperative percutaneous portal vein embolization: evaluation of adverse events in 188 patients. Radiology 2005;234:625–630.

22 De Baere T, Denys A, Madoff DC: Preoperative portal vein embolization: indications and technical considerations. Tech Vasc Interv Radiol 2007;10:67–78.

23 Denys A, Bize P, Demartines N, Deschamps F, De Baere T; Cardiovascular and Interventional Radiological Society of Europe: Quality improvement for portal vein embolization. Cardiovasc Intervent Radiol 2010;33:452–456.

24 Bruix J, Castells A, Bosch J, Feu F, Fuster J, Garcia-Pagan JC, Visa J, Bru C, Rodes J: Surgical resection of hepatocellular carcinoma in cirrhotic patients: prognostic value of preoperative portal pressure. Gastroenterology 1996;111:1018–1022.

25 Farges O, Malassagne B, Flejou JF, Balzan S, Sauvanet A, Belghiti J: Risk of major liver resection in patients with underlying chronic liver disease: a reappraisal. Ann Surg 1999;229:210–215.

26 Kusaka K, Imamura H, Tomiya T, Makuuchi M: Factors affecting liver regeneration after right portal vein embolization. Hepatogastroenterology 2004;51:532–535.

27 Madoff DC, Abdalla EK, Gupta S, Wu TT, Morris JS, Denys A, Wallace MJ, Morello FA, Jr., Ahrar K, Murthy R, Lunagomez S, Hicks ME, Vauthey JN: Transhepatic ipsilateral right portal vein embolization extended to segment IV: improving hypertrophy and resection outcomes with spherical particles and coils. J Vasc Interv Radiol 2005;16:215–225.

28 Giraudo G, Greget M, Oussoultzoglou E, Rosso E, Bachellier P, Jaeck D: Preoperative contralateral portal vein embolization before major hepatic resection is a safe and efficient procedure: a large single institution experience. Surgery 2008;143:476–482.

29 Kishi Y, Madoff DC, Abdalla EK, Palavecino M, Ribero D, Chun YS, Vauthey JN: Is embolization of segment 4 portal veins before extended right hepatectomy justified? Surgery 2008;144:744–751.

30 Schulte am Esch J, Schmelzle M, Fürst G, Robson SC, Krieg A, Duhme C, Tustas RY, Alexander A, Klein HM, Topp SA, Bode JG, Häussinger D, Eisenberger CF, Knoefel WT: Infusion of CD133+ bone marrow-derived stem cells after selective portal vein embolization enhances functional hepatic reserves after extended right hepatectomy: a retrospective single-center study. Ann Surg 2012;255:79–85.

31 Fürst G, Schulte am Esch J, Poll LW, Hosch SB, Fritz LB, Klein M, Godehardt E, Krieg A, Wecker B, Stoldt V, Stockschläder M, Eisenberger CF, Mödder U, Knoefel WT: Portal vein embolization and autologous CD133+ bone marrow stem cells for liver regeneration: initial experience. Radiology 2007;243:171–179.

32 Audollent R, Eveno C, Contreres JO, Hainaud P, Rampanou A, Dupuy E, Brouland JP, Pocard M: Bone marrow-derived endothelial and hematopoietic precursors cells enhance the metastasis of colon cancer in an orthotopic murine model. Int J Cancer 2011;129:2304–2305.

33 Olthof PB, Huisman F, Schaap FG, van Lienden KP, Bennink RJ, van Golen RF, Heger M, Verheij J, Jansen PL, Olde Damink SW, van Gulik TM: Effect of obeticholic acid on liver regeneration following portal vein embolization in an experimental model. Br J Surg 2017;104:590–599.

34 Beppu T, Nitta H, Hayashi H, Imai K, Okabe H, Nakagawa S, Hashimoto D, Chikamoto A, Ishiko T, Yoshida M, Yamashita Y, Baba H: Effect of branched-chain amino acid supplementation on functional liver regeneration in patients undergoing portal vein embolization and sequential hepatectomy: a randomized controlled trial. J Gastroenterol 2015;50:1197–1205.

35 Ogata S, Belghiti J, Farges O, Varma D, Sibert A, Vilgrain V: Sequential arterial and portal vein embolizations before right hepatectomy in patients with cirrhosis and hepatocellular carcinoma. Br J Surg 2006;93:1091–1098.

36 Aoki T, Imamura H, Hasegawa K, Matsukura A, Sano K, Sugawara Y, Kokudo N, Makuuchi M: Sequential preoperative arterial and portal venous embolizations in patients with hepatocellular carcinoma. Arch Surg 2004;139:766–774.

37 Kang BK, Kim JH, Kim KM, Ko GY, Yoon HK, Gwon DI, Sung KB: Transcatheter arterial chemoembolization for hepatocellular carcinoma after attempted portal vein embolization in 25 patients. AJR Am J Roentgenol 2009;193:W446–451.

38 Nagino M, Kanai M, Morioka A, Yamamoto H, Kawabata Y, Hayakawa N, Nimura Y: Portal and arterial embolization before extensive liver resection in patients with markedly poor functional reserve. J Vasc Interv Radiol 2000;11:1063–1068.

39 Inaba S, Takada T, Amano H, Yoshida M, Yamakawa Y, Yasuda H, Takada Y, Takeshita K, Koutake H, Takada K, Furui S, Hijikata H, Takada K: Combination of preoperative embolization of the right portal vein and hepatic artery prior to major hepatectomy in high-risk patients: a preliminary report. Hepatogastroenterology 2000;47:1077–1081.

40 Gruttadauria S, Luca A, Mandala L, Miraglia R, Gridelli B: Sequential preoperative ipsilateral portal and arterial embolization in patients with colorectal liver metastases. World J Surg 2006;30:576–578.

41 Yokoyama Y, Nagino M: Sequential PVE and TAE for biliary tract cancer and liver metastases; in Madoff DC, Makuuchi M, Mizuno T, Vauthey J-N (eds): Venous Embolization of the Liver. Radiologic and Surgical Practice. London, Springer, 2011.

42 Hwang S, Lee SG, Ko GY, Kim BS, Sung KB, Kim MH, Lee SK, Hong HN: Sequential preoperative ipsilateral hepatic vein embolization after portal vein embolization to induce further liver regeneration in patients with hepatobiliary malignancy. Ann Surg 2009;249:608–616.
43 Hwang S, Ha TY, Ko GY, Kwon DI, Song GW, Jung DH, Kim MH, Lee SK, Lee SG: Preoperative sequential portal and hepatic vein embolization in patients with hepatobiliary malignancy. World J Surg 2015;39:2990–2998.
44 Guiu B, Chevallier P, Denys A, Delhom E, Pierredon-Foulongne MA, Rouanet P, Fabre JM, Quenet F, Herrero A, Panaro F, Baudin G, Ramos J: Simultaneous trans-hepatic portal and hepatic vein embolization before major hepatectomy: the liver venous deprivation technique. Eur Radiol 2016;26:4259–4267.
45 Guiu B, Quenet F, Escal L, Bibeau F, Piron L, Rouanet P, Fabre JM, Jacquet E, Denys A, Kotzki PO, Verzilli D, Deshayes E: Extended liver venous deprivation before major hepatectomy induces marked and very rapid increase in future liver remnant function. Eur Radiol 2017;27:3343–3352.
46 Le Roy B, Perrey A, Fontarensky M, Gagniere J, Abergel A, Pereira B, Lambert C, Boyer L, Pezet D, Chabrot P, Buc E: Combined preoperative portal and hepatic vein embolization (biembolization) to improve liver regeneration before major liver resection: a preliminary report. World J Surg 2017;41:1848–1856.
47 Sparrelid E, Gilg S, Brismar TB, Lundell L, Isaksson B: Rescue ALPPS is efficient and safe after failed portal vein occlusion in patients with colorectal liver metastases. Langenbecks Arch Surg 2017;402:69–75.
48 Knoefel WT, Gabor I, Rehders A, Alexander A, Krausch M, Schulte am Esch J, Fürst G, Topp SA: In situ liver transection with portal vein ligation for rapid growth of the future liver remnant in two-stage liver resection. Br J Surg 2013;100:388–394.
49 Tschuor C, Croome KP, Sergeant G, Cano V, Schadde E, Ardiles V, Slankamenac K, Claria RS, de Santibanes E, Hernandez-Alejandro R, Clavien PA: Salvage parenchymal liver transection for patients with insufficient volume increase after portal vein occlusion – an extension of the ALPPS approach. Eur J Surg Oncol 2013;39:1230–1235.
50 Day RW, Conrad C, Vauthey JN, Aloia TA: Evaluating surgeon attitudes towards the safety and efficacy of portal vein occlusion and associating liver partition and portal vein ligation: a report of the MALINSA survey. HPB (Oxford) 2015;17:936–941.
51 Yamakado K, Takeda K, Matsumura K, Nakatsuka A, Hirano T, Kato N, Sakuma H, Nakagawa T, Kawarada Y: Regeneration of the un-embolized liver parenchyma following portal vein embolization. J Hepatol 1997;27:871–880.
52 Peng PD, Hyder O, Bloomston M, Marques H, Corona-Villalobos C, Dixon E, Pulitano C, Hirose K, Schulick RD, Barroso E, Aldrighetti L, Choti M, Shen F, Kamel I, Geschwind JF, Pawlik TM: Sequential intra-arterial therapy and portal vein embolization is feasible and safe in patients with advanced hepatic malignancies. HPB (Oxford) 2012;14:523–531.

Visceral Medicine

Review Article

Visc Med 2017;33:426–433
DOI: 10.1159/000479477

Published online: December 4, 2017

# Hypertrophy and Liver Function in ALPPS: Correlation with Morbidity and Mortality

Danby Kang[a] Erik Schadde[a–c]

[a]Department of Surgery, Rush University Medical Center, Chicago, IL, USA;
[b]Cantonal Hospital Winterthur, Winterthur, Switzerland;
[c]Institute of Physiology, Center for Integrative Human Physiology, University of Zurich, Zurich, Switzerland

**Keywords**

ALPPS · Liver function · Posthepatectomy liver failure

**Summary**

**Background:** ALPPS (associating liver partition and portal vein ligation for staged hepatectomy) was introduced with the promise to reduce posthepatectomy liver failure (PHLF) in extended hepatectomies but has higher morbidity and mortality rates compared to conventional methods of volume enhancement. There are few studies of the incidence of PHLF after ALPPS and little information on how to avoid PHLF by functional testing. It remains unclear what causes the compromise in liver function despite rapid volume gain and if any of the modifications proposed reduce the incidence of PHLF. This review summarizes published data on this topic. **Methods:** This is a systematic review that studies literature on the incidence of liver failure and assessment of liver function following ALPPS as well as modifications of the existing technique. Articles were searched in PubMed, evaluated, selected, and tabulated. **Results:** The literature search revealed 326 articles that met the selection criteria. PHLF criteria as defined by the International Study Group of Liver Surgery (ISGLS) were the most commonly used criteria, but PHLF was frequently not defined. PHLF occurred most frequently after stage 2 of ALPPS at around 30% in most larger studies. Hepatobiliary scintigraphy showed a discrepancy between volume and functional growth of the liver. Function increase was only 50% compared to volume increase. Mechanistic explanations using histologic analyses have been given to explain the immaturity of the liver after rapid hypertrophy. Modifications of ALPPS showed a comparable volumetric gain when compared to classic ALPPS, but data were lacking to assess PHLF. **Conclusion:** ALPPS has relatively high rates of PHLF, morbidity, and mortality. This may be explained by data demonstrating functional growth when compared to volume growth. ALPPS should not be performed without functional assessment and with caution.



## Introduction

The amount of liver that can be removed by liver resection is limited by the metabolic and functional capacity of the future liver remnant (FLR) after resection. The prospective postoperative functional liver capacity has for the longest time been quantified by the volume of this FLR as determined by cross-sectional imaging. Therefore, surgeons have developed strategies to increase the volume of the remnant liver by either minimizing the amount of liver resected [1], downsizing the mass to be resected, or increasing the FLR prior to resection by occlusion of the contralateral portal vein [2]. Volume increase after portal vein occlusion is by no means as fast as volume increase after liver resection proper. Data from live donor hepatectomy and standard liver resections show that the liver volume almost doubles within 10 days after hemi-hepatectomy [3]. In contrast, both surgical portal vein ligation (PVL) and portal vein embolization (PVE) require 3–6 weeks of waiting time and a re-evaluation before the tumor-involved portion can be safely resected [4]. The congruity of volume and function was never really challenged, except by some who considered whether PVE may have a larger impact on liver function beyond its modest impact on liver volume over time [5]. These authors must have felt that PVE increased the function of the FLR even if the volume only changed a little bit.



Erik Schadde, MD FACS FEBS (HPB)
Department of Surgery
Rush University Medical Center
1653 W. Congress Pkwy Jelke Building 7th Floor, 60612 Chicago, IL, USA
erik.schadde@uzh.ch

In 2012, Associating Liver Partition and Portal vein ligation for Staged hepatectomy (ALPPS) was introduced and reduced the 3–6 weeks waiting time while increasing the extent of FLR growth [6]. The procedure hailed a simultaneous deportalization and in-situ parenchymal transection to induce the same rapid liver growth that can be observed after liver resection proper and allowed the resection of extensive tumor masses in 2 stages in 1–2 weeks. The inaugural ALPPS report describes a median volumetric increase of 74% over a median of 9 days [6], and the first multicenter report of an international registry reported 81% volume increase over a median of 7 days [6, 7].

Initially, ALPPS was praised as the most important surgical innovation in liver surgery for years [8], because presumably it eliminated the fear of posthepatectomy liver failure (PHLF), the most common and the most feared complication of extended resections. However, the first analyses showed that ALPPS has a perioperative mortality of 9% and a complication rate of Clavien-Dindo > 3a of 40% [9]. This appears high when compared to 2-stage hepatectomies with a mortality of 3% and a major morbidity rate of 40% in a recent meta-analysis [10]. Lack of experience and the difficulty of the procedure served as an explanation for these disappointing outcomes of ALPPS [11]. However, when complications and mortality were dissected in a more granular fashion, it became obvious that 75% of the reported 90-day mortalities had to be attributed to PHLF and that liver failure criteria were present in 14% of patients even after stage 1 when no liver tissue had been resected yet [9]. Although it remained difficult to determine how much major morbidity is simply procedure-related and not actually caused by PHLF, this analysis raised the suspicion that ALPPS may in fact generate rapid volumetric growth without the congruent growth in liver function that is required for adequate postoperative recovery. It also appeared that there had been an over-reliance on liver volume when deciding whether patients can undergo stage-2 resection, and that rapidly grown livers are not made of the 'same material' as liver grown slowly after PVE. This concern has led some surgeons to routinely evaluate the function of the growing FLR rather than relying on volume assessment alone.

The purpose of this review is to summarize what we know about liver-related mortality and morbidity after ALPPS and to enumerate the studies that have attempted to shed light on the conundrum of volume and function in ALPPS. The review also investigates which mechanistic explanations have been presented to understand the functional deficiency of the rapidly volume-expanded liver in ALPPS. Finally, we ask if any of the proposed 'better' modifications of the ALPPS operation do not have the problem of functional deficiency of 'classic' ALPPS.

## Methods

PubMed was searched using the following algorithm: ((('ALPPS'(Title/Abstract) OR 'associating liver partition and portal vein ligation for staged hepatectomy'(Title/Abstract)) OR 'in situ split'(Title/Abstract)). A list of all references was made, and titles were screened. Studies that provided information on outcomes of ALPPS in terms of complication and mortality in relation to liver function following ALPPS were selected for abstract review. Additionally, all studies examining liver function tests to guide resection in ALPPS as well as mechanistic studies to better understand the volume-function relationship were evaluated in abstract format. Modifications of ALPPS and their outcomes were reviewed. Language was restricted to English. Opinion, editorials, letters, and commentary were excluded. Single case reports and technical letters that were deemed highly relevant to our review were included, given the emerging nature of the topic. There was no restriction on study types. Several studies were excluded based on the full text review.

After selection, articles were grouped under 4 topics:

- Liver-related morbidity and mortality after ALPPS.
- Interstage liver function in ALPPS.
- Mechanisms proposed to explain the lack of congruence of volume and function.
- Impact of modifications of ALPPS on the volume/function dilemma.

## Results

*Literature Review Results*

Figure 1 shows the review and selection process. 326 references were initially identified and 58 abstracts reviewed. A total of 29 full text articles were selected for the review.

*Incidence of Liver Failure and Higher Complications after ALPPS*

A total of 18 studies reported major complications and mortality after ALPPS and related those findings to postoperative liver function and PHLF (table 1). The most common criteria used in defining PHLF were the liver failure criteria of the International Study Group of Liver Surgery (ISGLS) [12], followed by the 50-50 criteria [13]. The peak bilirubin criterion [14] was used in only 2 studies. 7 of the listed studies employed more than one criterion to evaluate PHLF. 3 studies did not specify the criteria used. The incidence of PHLF after ALPPS using any combination of the three criteria ranged from 8 to 36% with the majority of larger studies demonstrating a rate of around 30%. Perioperative complications were reported using the Clavien-Dindo grading system [15] in all but 2 studies. Clinically significant morbidity after ALPPS was 13–44% and 14–36% for grades 3a or higher and 3b or higher, respectively. 1 study demonstrated no mortality and a very low morbidity but reported a 29% rate of ISGLS-defined liver failure. Only 1 study examined how many mortalities after ALPPS were likely due to PHLF by analyzing the causes of 28 mortalities in 320 patients. The study showed that up to 75% of all mortalities after ALPPS were likely a consequence of PHLF. It was also shown that PHLF by ISGLS criteria after stage 1 and a MELD (Model for End-stage Liver Disease) score > 10 prior to stage 2 were significant risk factors for 90-day mortality after ALPPS, while standardized FLR volume prior to stage 2 or experience of the center performing ALPPS

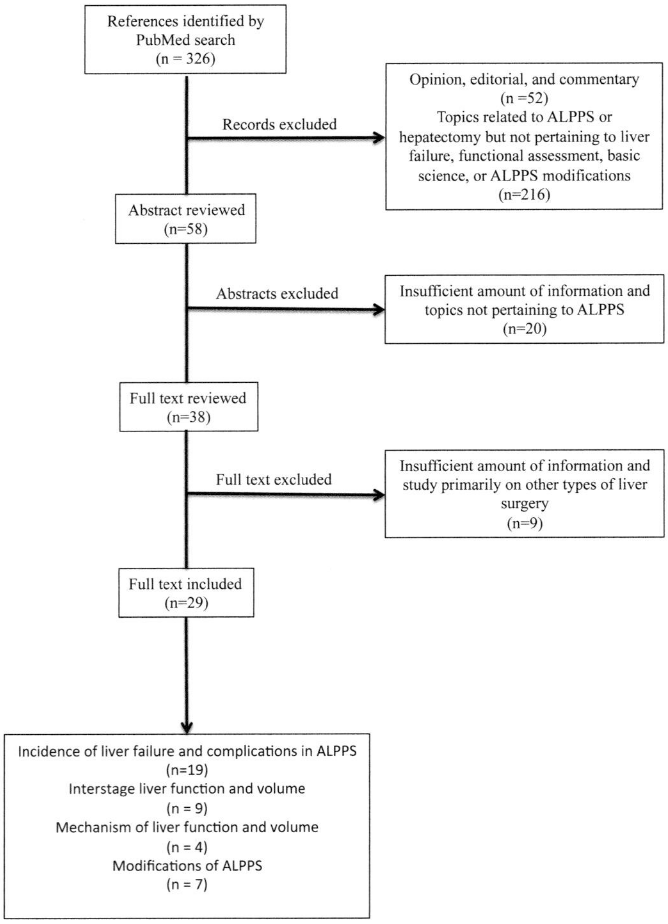


**Fig. 1.** Flowchart of databases searched, the strategy used, and exclusions performed.

were not [9]. A correlation between FLR volume and complications did not exist. Next to MELD score or ISGLS criteria after stage 1, kinetic growth rate of the FLR [16] and a dedicated ALPPS futility score [17] have been proposed to assess the risk of stage-2 resection.

*Assessment of Interstage Liver Function*

Table 2 lists the 5 studies investigating interstage liver function assessment. So far, hepatobiliary scintigraphy (HBS) has been the test of choice due to its ability to selectively evaluate regions of the liver for function. Early reports evaluated only the proportion of HIDA (hepatobiliary iminodiacetic acid scan) signal coming from the FLR as a percentage of the total HIDA signal prior to stage 2 [18]. Since this approach yielded no information about total function of the liver, it was generally abandoned by most. Later studies used an uptake index derived from an analysis of HIDA uptake from the blood pool in the first 5 min, as established by the Amsterdam group [19]. There are only 2 studies in ALPPS so far using this methodology [20, 21]. These studies, including 10 and 28 patients, respectively, showed that functional increase was less (28 and 29% over 6 and 7 days, respectively) than volume increase (57 and 78% over 6 and 8 days, respectively). ICG-R15 (indocyanine green retention rate at 15 min) is a global liver function test based on the proportion of remaining ICG after intravenous (i.v.) injection after 15 min and was used in 2 studies. One study showed ICG-R15 decreased from 9.9 to 7% between stages but increased to 33% after stage 2 [21]. Another study showed an increase from 3.6 to 5.4% postoperatively [16]. LiMAx (maximum liver function capacity) is another global liver function test based on hepatic enzyme metabolism, which is quantified using a breath test after i.v. methacetin has been administered. It has so far only been published in 1 single case report which demonstrated a dramatic decrease in global liver function between stage-1 and stage-2 ALPPS [42].

*Investigations into the Mechanism of Function and Volume*

A total of 5 studies addressed the potential mechanism of the function/volume question after ALPPS (table 3). A first effort was directed at making sure that the volume increase measured with volumetry in ALPPS is not just edema or regenerative steatosis by using functional magnetic resonance imaging (MRI) data. It was concluded that volume increase after ALPPS is indeed cellular proliferation and not edema or steatosis according to MRI [23]. A second study came to the same conclusion [24].

Matsuo et al. [25] focused their investigation on histology specimens from patients undergoing ALPPS. Histology, electron microscopy, and immunohistochemistry staining showed findings consistent with immature hepatocytes. In a second study, immunohistochemistry and electron-microscopy of bile duct canaliculi showed weaker MDR1 staining, immature microvilli, and leaky tight junctions, despite an adequate quantity of bile duct canaliculi overall [26].

*Modifications of ALPPS*

A total of 7 studies on 6 different modification techniques were reviewed (table 4). Volume increase in ALPPS modification studies ranged from 53 to 76%. PHLF was reported at 13.6% in only 1 study [27]. The remaining studies reported no liver failure. However, in the majority of the studies, the criteria used to define PHLF were not specified. There was no information on liver function based on HBS, ICG, or LiMAx.

## Discussion

This review gives a first synopsis of data published on the volume/function problem to explain the high morbidity and mortality after the novel ALPPS procedure. It points to the available evidence that liver failure and major complications after ALPPS are higher than would be expected with the extensive increase in liver volume. It supports the claim that the high liver failure rate despite increase in volume is likely due to an intrinsic functional defect following rapid hypertrophy in classic ALPPS. This results in uncertainty as to when to progress to resection after ALPPS stage 1 has been performed. The mechanistic understanding of why rapid hypertrophy fails to provide some patients with adequate liver function despite increases in volume is still preliminary, and so far there is no data to conclude that the new ALPPS modifications proposed are helpful to overcome the volume-function problem of rapid hypertrophy.

**Tab. 1.** Incidence of liver failure and complications after ALPPS

| Author [ref.] | Year | n | Criteria for liver failure | PHLF after stage 1, n (%) | PHLF after stage 2, n (%) | Clavien grade 3a or higher, n (%) | Clavien grade 3b or higher, n (%) | Liver-related mortality[a], n (%) |
|---|---|---|---|---|---|---|---|---|
| Linecker [17] | 2016 | 47 vs. 481[b] | ISGLS | 10 (23) vs.<br>36 (9) | NR | NR | 15 (33) vs.<br>30 (7) | 17/45 (36) |
| Schadde [9] | 2015 | 320 | ISGLS<br>50-50<br>Bili > 7[c] | 44 (14)<br>4 (1)<br>5 (2) | 93 (30)<br>27 (9)<br>21 (7) | NR | NR | 21/28 (75) |
| Schadde [28] | 2014 | 202 | 50-50 | 16 (9) | | 80 (40) | 56 (28) | 8/19 (42) |
| Truant [36] | 2015 | 62 | 50-50 | 3 (5) | 15 (25) | 25 (40) | NR | 3/8 (38) |
| Olthof [20] | 2016 | 60 | ISGLS[d] | 1 (2) | 5 (8) | 24 (40) | NR | 2/4 (50) |
| Schadde [7] | 2014 | 48 | 50-50 | 0 | 6 (13) | NR | 13 (27) | NR |
| Kambakamba [16] | 2016 | 36 | ISGLS<br>50-50 | NR<br>NR | 13 (36)<br>8 (22) | NR | 13 (36) | NR |
| Alvarez [18] | 2015 | 30 | ISGL + 50-50 | 0 | 4 (13) | 13 (43) | 9 (31) | 0 |
| Wanis [37] | 2017 | 30 | ISGLS<br>50-50 | 2 (7)<br>0 | 8 (31)<br>1 (4) | NR | 8 (26) | 0 |
| Serenari [30] | 2017 | 20 | Bili > 7<br>all 3[d] | 1 (5)<br>0 | 1 (5)<br>3 (15) | 5 (25)[d] | NR | 1/1 (100) |
| Alvarez [38] | 2013 | 15 | ISGLS | 3 (20) | | 5 (33) | 4 (27) | 0 |
| Hernandez-Alejandro [39] | 2015 | 14 | ISGLS + 50-50 | 4 (29) | | NR | 2 (14) | 0 |
| Tanaka [34] | 2015 | 11 | ISGLS | 2 (18) | 4 (36) | 4 (36) | 2 (18) | 0 |
| Sala [40] | 2012 | 10 | ISGLS | 2 (20) | | 2 (20) | 0 | 0 |
| Li [41] | 2013 | 9 | ISGLS | 0 | 2 (22) | 2 (22) | 3 (33) | 0 |
| Vivarelli [42] | 2015 | 9 | 50-50 | 0 | 1 (11.1) | 4 (44.4) | NR | 1/1 (100) |
| Ratti [43] | 2014 | 8 | ISGLS + 50-50 | 1 (13) | 0 | 3 (38) | 1 (13) | 0 |
| Matsuo [25] | 2016 | 8 | ISGLS | 2 (25) | | 1 (13) | NR | 0 |
| Matsuo [26] | 2017 | 8 | ISGLS<br>50-50 | 3 (37.5)<br>0 | | 3 (37.5) | NR | 0 |

[a]Liver-related mortality is the percent of 90-day mortality.
[b]Numbers reported as futile vs. non-futile operations in the study.
[c]Peak bilirubin criterion was modified in this study to reflect bilirubin > 7 mg/dl on postoperative day 5 due to data availability.
[d]ISGLS grade A was excluded in these studies.
PHLF = Posthepatectomy liver failure; ISGLS = International Study Group of Liver Surgery definition of liver failure according to Rahbari et al. [29]; 50-50: fifty/fifty criterion for liver failure according to Balzan et al. [13]; Bili > 7 = bilirubin > 7 mg/dl according to Mullen et al. [14]; NR = not reported.

Very few reports on ALPPS analyzed the morbidity and mortality under the aspect of whether they are actually caused by PHLF, the very reason why regenerative maneuvers like PVE, PVL, or ALPPS are performed in extended liver resection to start with. Curiously, studies on ALPPS do not report PHLF using any of the common metrics in their analyses. The 2 studies that dissected out morbidity and mortality after ALPPS in larger cohorts beyond established severity gradings and typing of complications came to the conclusion that the vast majority of complications is due to PHLF despite adequate liver volumes prior to stage 2 [9, 28]. The first registry analysis showed that of the 19/202 patients with 90-day mortality, 8 patients were judged to have liver failure by their clinicians and the incidence of liver failure by 50-50 criteria in all patients was 9% [28]. The second registry analysis focused entirely on mortality and showed that 21/28 (75%) mortalities were caused by liver failure and that 32% of all patients had liver failure using any of three criteria (ISGLS, 50-50, and peak bilirubin > 7 mg/dl). 20% of patients with liver failure died within 90 days after ALPPS [9].

Because PHLF presents in so many different ways, it remains difficult to attribute complications incurred to liver failure without formally assessing at least some to the accepted liver failure criteria based on postoperative laboratory values of INR (international normalized ratio) and total bilirubin at postoperative day 5 and beyond [13, 14, 29]. Meticulous reports on liver failure criteria should therefore be encouraged for any future reports on ALPPS outcomes. It is interesting to note that liver failure by ISGLS criteria in published series is only 8.3% [20] or 15% [30] in the 2 series in which HBS was performed to guide clinical management, and 36% in a series [16] in which no HBS was used. It suggests that clinical management with HBS may be able to avoid liver failure after ALPPS.

Interestingly, outcomes after ALPPS in the registry studies are very similar to outcomes reported for a contemporary series of 285 extended hepatectomies in an experienced liver resection center. Only 23% of these extended hepatectomies had preoperative PVE to increase the size of the FLR [31]. There was an incidence of PHLF of 28% and a mortality rate of 9%, and 84% of these mortali-

**Tab. 2.** Assessment of interstage liver function in relation to volume

| Author [ref.] | Year | n | Baseline function assessment | Interstage functional assessment | | | | | | | | | Functional increase[a], % | Volume increase, % | Days between stages, n |
|---|---|---|---|---|---|---|---|---|---|---|---|---|---|---|---|
| | | | | ISGLS after stage 1 | ICG | HBS % of counts | HBS AI, %/min/m$^2$ | HBS HIBA, % | LiMAx | MELD | functional KGR, %/day | volume KGR, %/day | | | |
| Linecker [17] | 2016 | 47 vs. 481[b] | 7 vs. 6 MELD) | yes | NR | NR | NR | NR | NR | 11 vs. 8 | NR | NR | NR | 77 vs. 70 | 5 |
| Schadde [9] | 2015 | 320 | NR | yes | NR | NR | NR | NR | NR | >10[c] | NR | NR | NR | NR | 14 |
| Olthof [20] | 2017 | 60 | 3.7 (AI)[d] | yes | NR | 40.4 | 5.5[d] | NR | NR | NR | NR | NR | 29 | 78 | 7–8 |
| Kambakamba [16] | 2016 | 36 | 3.6 (ICG-R15) 22.3 (ICG-PDR) | yes | 5.4 (R15) 20.2 (PDR) | NR | NR | NR | NR | NR | NR | 6.9 | NR | 53.7 | 6 |
| Alvarez [18] | 2015 | 30 | NR | yes | NR | 41 | NR | NR | NR | NR | NR | 13.8 | NR | 90 | 6 |
| Serenari[e] [30] | 2017 | 20 | NR | yes | NR | 30 vs. 41 | 0.94 vs. 2.07 | 13 vs. 23 | NR | NR | NR | NR | NR | NR | 6 |
| Tanaka [34] | 2015 | 10 | NR | yes | NR | 47.6 | NR | NR | NR | NR | NR | NR | 52 | 54 | 7 |
| Sparrelid [21] | 2017 | 9 | 9.9 (ICG-R15) 1.8 (AI) 25.3 (% of counts) | NR | 7 (R15) | 33.9 | 2.6 | NR | NR | NR | 4.7 | 9.4 | 28 | 57 | 6 |
| Oldhafer [22] | 2016 | 1 | 282 (LiMAx) | NR | NR | NR | NR | NR | 245 then 371 | NR | NR | NR | −13 (LiMAx) then +31 | 60 then 82 | 7 then 11 |

[a]Based on hepatobiliary scintigraphy, with the exception of the study using LiMAx.
[b]Numbers reported as futile vs. non-futile operations in the study.
[c]MELD > 10 indicates increased risk of 90-day mortality.
[d]Amsterdam index was modified in this study to be expressed as %/min. Body surface area was not used in the calculation.
[e]Results were provided as patients with liver failure vs. no liver failure. Combined results could not be calculated with the given data.
ISGLS = Post-resection liver failure criteria of the International Study Group for Liver Surgery; ICG = indocyanine green; ICG-R15 = indocyanine green clearance measured as plasma retention at 15 min (%); ICG-PDR = indocyanine green plasma disappearance rate (%/min); HBS = hepatobiliary scintigraphy; uptake in % = future liver remnant (FLR) function calculated by radioactivity count of FLR divided by total liver radioactivity count (%); AI = Amsterdam Index calculated using uptake kinetics between 150 and 350 s in %/min/m2 as described by Dinant et al. [35]; HIBA = Hospital Italiano de Buenos Aires index calculated by multiplying total liver uptake between 150 and 350 s by uptake in % according to Serenari et al. [30]; LiMAx = liver maximum function capacity test based on hepatocyte metabolism (μg/h/kg); MELD = Model for End-Stage Liver Disease; KGR = kinetic growth rate (%/day); NR = not reported.

**Tab. 3.** Investigations into the mechanism of function and volume in ALPPS

| Author [ref.] | Year | n | Subject | Method | Findings |
|---|---|---|---|---|---|
| Eshmuminov [23] | 2017 | 16 | hepatocyte proliferation | human histology MRI | no increased steatosis or cellular edema |
| Olthof [44] | 2016 | 12 | functional vs. volume growth in rabbits after ALPPS | HBS | volume but no functional increase when compared to PVE in rabbits |
| Sheng [24] | 2017 | 10 | hepatocyte proliferation | DKI IHC | true liver hypertrophy in ALPPS |
| Matsuo [25] | 2016 | 8 | hepatocyte maturity | human histology IHC electron microscopy | immaturity of hepatocytes |
| Matsuo [26] | 2017 | 8 | bile duct canaliculi network maturity | human histology IHC electron microscopy | structurally and functionally immature bile canalicular network |

MRI = Magnetic resonance imaging; HBS = hepatobiliary scintigraphy; PVE = portal vein embolization; DKI = diffusion kurtosis imaging; IHC = immunohistochemistry.

ties fulfilled ISGLS criteria for liver failure. In contrast, a recent meta-analysis on outcomes after 459 2-stage hepatectomies for colorectal liver metastases reported a mortality rate of only 3% and a major complication rate of 40% without further information on liver failure criteria [10]. The 2-stage hepatectomy approach with the regenerative liver surgery maneuvers of PVE and PVL should improve the morbidity and mortality of extended resections. Given these data, it is fair to conclude that ALPPS has the same risk of liver failure, mortality, and complications incurred by extended resection and does not seem to reduce this risk.

The most important practical question in clinical ALPPS management is how to assess function and volume prior to proceeding to stage-2 resection. The overarching problem in the field of measuring liver function in ALPPS remains that HBS so far appears to be the only available tool to measure regional liver function in the western world [32] but there is no standardized methodology of HBS that is easily reproducible. Despite this, all 5 studies using HBS in ALPPS, including 1 case report [33], converge on the fact that while there is some increase in liver function in the FLR after ALPPS, the functional increase is always less than the volume increase between stage 1 and stage 2 (table 2). Most worrisome are the 2 studies that use HBS uptake kinetics to quantify regional liver function (also called the 'Amsterdam index'). Both studies come to the conclusion that the functional increase of the FLR after ALPPS is only 37% [20] or 49% [31] of the volume increase, respectively. Such findings indicate that volume, currently the principal determinant for progression to the second stage, overestimates the function of the FLR by up to 50%, which may easily explain the high incidence of liver failure despite adequate volume. In the study of 27 patients with paired measurements, only 7 patients achieved an increase in liver function in their FLR beyond 50%, and 4 of these patients took more than 7 days to get beyond 50% function [20].

In the first reports, HBS was quantified by giving the proportion of scintigraphic signal that can be captured during the uptake phase or during the entire scan from the FLR and the portal vein-deprived side [18]. The downside of this '% of counts' technique is that it does not indicate a drop in liver function in case the overall liver function decreases. It simply provides clinicians with a proportion of total function without quantifying total function. The study that reported a volume increase of 52% with a functional increase of 54% used this methodology and appears to indicate a congruence of volume and function increase [34].

In contrast, the Amsterdam group has long ago developed a method to derive liver function from uptake kinetics between 150 and 350 s after injection using the HBS scan, and established their index for liver function expressed as uptake per min per $m^2$ [32]. Based on a series of liver resections, it has been shown that 2.7%/min/$m^2$ likely represents adequate liver function to master metabolic demands after resection [35]. An initial case report of this methodology in ALPPS [33] and a subsequent study using this methodology showed an astonishing functional deficit of the rapidly volume-increased liver [20].

The 2 studies with paired measurements prior to stage 1 and prior to stage 2 had too few outcome events to allow a solid C-statistic to determine a cut-off for preoperative liver function for the FLR [20, 31]. Studies with no paired measurements before and after stage 1 are not able to provide information on the effect of rapid hypertrophy on function changes [30], but they may provide information on when to proceed with stage 2 based on functional data. The Buenos Aires group attempted to develop a cut-off, but unfortunately they invented a new HBS metrics model, the 'Hospital Italiano of Buenos Aires (HIBA)' score, which makes their results difficult to compare to other uptake kinetics data published so far and difficult to reproduce for other centers [30]. Although there appears to be an emerging consensus among many groups that ALPPS should not be performed without HBS regional liver function tests prior to stage 2, the newly developed HIBA score cut-off of 15% has to first be validated by other centers.

Of course the lack of congruence of volume and function after ALPPS has to be explained mechanistically. The first concern

**Tab. 4.** Modifications of ALPPS and available data on liver failure and function

| Author [ref.] | Year | n | Modification | Volume increase, % | PHLF, n (%) | PHLF criteria used | Clavien-Dindo grade 3a or higher, n (%) | Clavien-Dindo grade 3b or higher, n (%) |
|---|---|---|---|---|---|---|---|---|
| Robles [27] | 2016 | 22 | ALTPS | 61 | 3 (14) | NR | NR | NR |
| Wang [45] | 2017 | 10 | RALPPS | 53 | 0 | NR | NR | 2 (20) |
| Petrowsky [46] | 2015 | 6 | p-ALPPS | 60 | 0 | NR | NR | 2 (33) |
| Gall [47] | 2014 | 5 | RALPPS | 62 | 0 | NR | 0 | 0 |
| De Santibanes [48] | 2016 | 4 | Mini ALPPS | 63 | 0 | 50-50 | NR | NR |
| Peng[a] [49] | 2016 | 4 | TBPVE | 66 | NR | NR | NR | NR |
| Li [50] | 2014 | 2 | Hybrid ALPPS | 76 | 0 | NR | 1 (50) | NR |

[a]Full text paper was not available in English; abstract was published in English and was used for data.
PHLF = Posthepatectomy liver failure; ALTPS = Associating Liver Tourniquet with Portal vein ligation for Staged hepatectomy: modification of ALPPS where a tourniquet is used to obliterate the flow between the portal vein-supplied and the portal vein-deprived part of the liver; RALPPS = radiofrequency-assisted ALPPS where transection is replaced by radiofrequency ablation; p-ALPPS = partial ALPPS where only partial transection is performed instead of complete transection; TBPVE = terminal branches portal vein embolization, a variation of PVE pioneered in China; NR = not reported.

raised was that the rapid and extensive volume increase in ALPPS is not true cellular proliferation of functioning hepatocytes, but interstitial edema or intracellular fat accumulation/regenerative steatosis. 2 MRI studies, 1 in patients and 1 in rats, have now debunked this concern [23, 34]. Both studies show convincingly that ALPPS induces true cellular proliferation.

Interestingly, both hepatocytes and bile duct canaliculi, however, displayed characteristics of immaturity in histology [25, 26]. Whether these deficiencies are a transient or permanent defect of rapid hypertrophy has yet to be determined. The studies suggest that progressing to stage 2 within a week may be premature despite the impressive volumetric increase.

It may well be that the problem with liver function is an intrinsic problem only for classic ALPPS, and that the modified ALPPS approaches overcome the problem of volume/function. Unfortunately, the reports on ALPPS modifications report on very small series of patients and are generally limited to demonstrating a volume increase as large as that seen in classic ALPPS. The main focus of these reports seems to be to develop less invasive procedures based on the assumption that the complications of ALPPS stem largely from surgical severity and lack of experience of the surgeons. Functional studies of the FLR have not been added to these reports on modifications, and the awareness of the volume/function problem is limited. At this stage, reports on modifications should carefully address PHLF or, even better, evaluate liver function before and after ALPPS using metrics like HBS, LiMAx, or ICG.

The limitations of this review are primarily the small number of published studies in an emerging field as well as the small sample size in each study. It also appears that clinicians reporting on their experience with ALPPS have only limited access to liver function tests such as HBS, LiMAx, or ICG. There also remains the concern of a reporting bias across all the small uncontrolled series, especially the reports from the voluntary international ALPPS registry which has not been subject to independent monitoring or audit.

## Conclusion

In summary, ALPPS has a high incidence of liver failure caused by a discrepancy between volumetric growth and functional increase of the FLR, which is alarming and needs to be better understood. Direct measurement of regional liver function may protect from liver failure after stage 2, but there is no consensus on reliable metrics. So far, there is no proof that efforts to improve ALPPS by modifications are effective to address this problem. Until these questions are addressed, ALPPS should be considered to be an experimental procedure and only be used in a highly controlled research environment.

## Disclosure Statement

The authors do not have a conflict of interest for this article.

## References

1 Jarnagin WR, Gonen M, Fong Y, et al: Improvement in perioperative outcome after hepatic resection: analysis of 1,803 consecutive cases over the past decade. Ann Surg 2002;236:397–406, discussion 406–397.

2 Van Lienden KP, van den Esschert JW, de Graaf W, et al: Portal vein embolization before liver resection: a systematic review. Cardiovasc Intervent Radiol 2013; 36:25–34.

3 Nadalin S, Testa G, Malago M, et al: Volumetric and functional recovery of the liver after right hepatectomy for living donation. Liver Transpl 2004;10:1024–1029.

4 Abulkhir A, Limongelli P, Healey AJ, et al: Preoperative portal vein embolization for major liver resection: a meta-analysis. Ann Surg 2008;247:49–57.
5 Farges O, Belghiti J, Kianmanesh R, et al: Portal vein embolization before right hepatectomy: prospective clinical trial. Ann Surg 2003;237:208–217.
6 Schnitzbauer AA, Lang SA, Goessmann H, et al: Right portal vein ligation combined with in situ splitting induces rapid left lateral liver lobe hypertrophy enabling 2-staged extended right hepatic resection in small-for-size settings. Ann Surg 2012;255:405–414.
7 Schadde E, Ardiles V, Slankamenac K, et al: ALPPS offers a better chance of complete resection in patients with primarily unresectable liver tumors compared with conventional-staged hepatectomies: results of a multicenter analysis. World J Surg 2014;38:1510–1519.
8 De Santibanes E, Clavien PA: Playing Play-Doh to prevent postoperative liver failure: the 'ALPPS' approach. Ann Surg 2012;255:415–417.
9 Schadde E, Raptis DA, Schnitzbauer AA, et al: Prediction of mortality after ALPPS stage-1: an analysis of 320 patients from the International ALPPS Registry. Ann Surg 2015;262:780–785, discussion 785–786.
10 Lam VW, Laurence JM, Johnston E, et al: A systematic review of two-stage hepatectomy in patients with initially unresectable colorectal liver metastases. HPB (Oxford) 2013;15:483–491.
11 Lang H, de Santibanes E, Clavien PA: Outcome of ALPPS for perihilar cholangiocarcinoma: case-control analysis including the first series from the international ALPPS registry. HPB (Oxford) 2017;19:379–380.
12 Rahbari NN, Reissfelder C, Koch M, et al: The predictive value of postoperative clinical risk scores for outcome after hepatic resection: a validation analysis in 807 patients. Ann Surg Oncol 2011;18:3640–3649.
13 Balzan S, Belghiti J, Farges O, et al: The '50-50 criteria' on postoperative day 5: an accurate predictor of liver failure and death after hepatectomy. Ann Surg 2005; 242:824–828, discussion 828–829.
14 Mullen JT, Ribero D, Reddy SK, et al: Hepatic insufficiency and mortality in 1,059 noncirrhotic patients undergoing major hepatectomy. J Am Coll Surg 2007; 204:854–862, discussion 862–854.
15 Dindo D, Demartines N, Clavien PA: Classification of surgical complications. Ann Surg 2004;240:205–213.
16 Kambakamba P, Stocker D, Reiner CS, et al: Liver kinetic growth rate predicts postoperative liver failure after ALPPS. HPB (Oxford) 2016;18:800–805.
17 Linecker M, Stavrou GA, Oldhafer KJ, et al: The ALPPS risk score: avoiding futile use of ALPPS. Ann Surg 2016;264:763–771.
18 Alvarez FA, Ardiles V, de Santibanes M, et al: Associating liver partition and portal vein ligation for staged hepatectomy offers high oncological feasibility with adequate patient safety: a prospective study at a single center. Ann Surg 2015;261:723–732.
19 De Graaf W, Vetelainen RL, de Bruin K, et al: 99m Tc-GSA scintigraphy with SPECT for assessment of hepatic function and functional volume during liver regeneration in a rat model of partial hepatectomy. J Nucl Med 2008;49:122–128.
20 Olthof PB, Tomassini F, Huespe P, et al: Hepatobiliary scintigraphy to evaluate liver function in ALPPS: liver volume overestimates liver function. Surgery 2017;162: 775–783.
21 Sparrelid E, Jonas E, Tzortzakakis A, et al: Dynamic evaluation of liver volume and function in associating liver partition and portal vein ligation for staged hepatectomy. J Gastrointest Surg 2017;21:967–974.
22 Oldhafer F, Ringe KI, Timrott K, et al: Monitoring of liver function in a 73-year old patient undergoing 'Associating Liver Partition and Portal vein ligation for Staged hepatectomy': case report applying the novel liver maximum function capacity test. Patient Saf Surg 2016;10:16.
23 Eshmuminov D, Tschuor C, Raptis DA, Boss A, et al: Rapid liver volume increase induced by associating liver partition with portal vein ligation for staged hepatectomy (ALPPS): is it edema, steatosis, or true proliferation? Surgery 2017;161:1549–1552.
24 Sheng RF, Wang HQ, Jin KP, et al: Histogram analyses of diffusion kurtosis indices and apparent diffusion coefficient in assessing liver regeneration after ALPPS and a comparative study with portal vein ligation. J Magn Reson Imaging 2017;DOI: 10.1002/jmri.25793.
25 Matsuo K, Murakami T, Kawaguchi D, et al: Histologic features after surgery associating liver partition and portal vein ligation for staged hepatectomy versus those after hepatectomy with portal vein embolization. Surgery 2016;159:1289–1298.
26 Matsuo K, Hiroshima Y, Yamazaki K, et al.: Immaturity of bile canalicular-ductule networks in the future liver remnant while associating liver partition and portal vein occlusion for staged hepatectomy (ALPPS). Ann Surg Oncol 2017;24:2456–2464.
27 Robles R, Parrilla P, Lopez-Conesa A, et al: Tourniquet modification of the associating liver partition and portal ligation for staged hepatectomy procedure. Br J Surg 2014;101:1129–1134, discussion 1134.
28 Schadde E, Ardiles V, Robles-Campos R, et al: Early survival and safety of ALPPS: first report of the International ALPPS Registry. Ann Surg 2014;260:829–836, discussion 836–828.
29 Rahbari NN, Garden OJ, Padbury R, et al: Posthepatectomy liver failure: a definition and grading by the International Study Group of Liver Surgery (ISGLS). Surgery 2011;149:713–724.
30 Serenari M, Collaud C, Alvarez FA, et al: Interstage assessment of remnant liver function in ALPPS using hepatobiliary scintigraphy: prediction of posthepatectomy liver failure and introduction of the HIBA index. Ann Surg 2017;DOI: 10.1097/SLA.0000000000002150.
31 Truant S, El Amrani M, Skrzypczyk C, et al: Factors associated with fatal liver failure after extended hepatectomy. HPB (Oxford) 2017;19:682–687.
32 Olthof PB, van Gulik TM, Bennink RJ: Optimal use of hepatobiliary scintigraphy before liver resection. HPB (Oxford) 2016;18:870.
33 Cieslak KP, Olthof PB, van Lienden KP, et al: Assessment of liver function using $^{99m}$Tc-mebrofenin hepatobiliary scintigraphy in ALPPS (associating liver partition and portal vein ligation for staged hepatectomy). Case Rep Gastroenterol 2015;9:353–360.
34 Tanaka K, Matsuo K, Murakami T, et al: Associating liver partition and portal vein ligation for staged hepatectomy (ALPPS): short-term outcome, functional changes in the future liver remnant, and tumor growth activity. Eur J Surg Oncol 2015;41:506–512.
35 Dinant S, de Graaf W, Verwer BJ, et al: Risk assessment of posthepatectomy liver failure using hepatobiliary scintigraphy and CT volumetry. J Nucl Med 2007; 48:685–692.
36 Truant S, Scatton O, Dokmak S, et al: Associating liver partition and portal vein ligation for staged hepatectomy (ALPPS): impact of the inter-stages course on morbi-mortality and implications for management. Eur J Surg Oncol 2015;41:674–682.
37 Wanis KN, Buac S, Linecker M, et al: Patient survival after simultaneous ALPPS and colorectal resection. World J Surg 2017;41:1119–1125.
38 Alvarez FA, Ardiles V, Sanchez Claria R, et al: Associating liver partition and portal vein ligation for staged hepatectomy (ALPPS): tips and tricks. J Gastrointest Surg 2013;17:814–821.
39 Hernandez-Alejandro R, Bertens KA, Pineda-Solis K, Croome KP: Can we improve the morbidity and mortality associated with the associating liver partition with portal vein ligation for staged hepatectomy (ALPPS) procedure in the management of colorectal liver metastases? Surgery 2015;157:194–201.
40 Sala S, Ardiles V, Ulla M, et al: Our initial experience with ALPPS technique: encouraging results. Updates Surg 2012;64:167–172.
41 Li J, Girotti P, Königsrainer I, et al: ALPPS in right trisectionectomy: a safe procedure to avoid postoperative liver failure? J Gastrointest Surg 2013;17:956–961.
42 Vivarelli M, Vincenzi P, Montalti R, et al: ALPPS procedure for extended liver resections: a single centre experience and a systematic review. PloS One 2015; 10:e0144019.
43 Ratti F, Cipriani F, Gagliano A, et al: Defining indications to ALPPS procedure: technical aspects and open issues. Updates Surg 2014;66:41–49.
44 Olthof PB, Schadde E, van Lienden KP, et al: Hepatic parenchymal transection increases liver volume but not function after portal vein embolization in rabbits. Surgery 2017;162:732–741.
45 Wang Q, Yan J, Feng X, et al: Safety and efficacy of radiofrequency-assisted ALPPS (RALPPS) in patients with cirrhosis-related hepatocellular carcinoma. Int J Hyperthermia 2017;33:846–852.
46 Petrowsky H, Gyori G, de Oliveira M, et al: Is partial-ALPPS safer than ALPPS? A single-center experience. Ann Surg 2015;261:e90–92.
47 Gall TM, Sodergren MH, Frampton AE, et al: Radiofrequency-assisted Liver Partition with Portal vein ligation (RALPP) for liver regeneration. Ann Surg 2015; 261:e45–46.
48 De Santibanes E, Alvarez FA, Ardiles V, et al: Inverting the ALPPS paradigm by minimizing first stage impact: the Mini-ALPPS technique. Langenbecks Arch Surg 2016;401:557–563.
49 Peng SY, Huang CY, Li JT, et al: Terminal branches portal vein embolization for planed hepatectomy (Article in Chinese). Zhonghua Wai Ke Za Zhi 2016;54: 664–668.
50 Li J, Kantas A, Ittrich H, et al: Avoid 'all-touch' by hybrid ALPPS to achieve oncological efficacy. Ann Surg 2016;263:e6–7.

# Imprint

**ISSN Print Edition:** 2297–4725
**ISSN Online Edition:** 2297–475X

**Journal Homepage:** http://www.karger.com/vis

**Publication Data:** Volume 33, 2017 of 'Visceral Medicine' appears with 6 issues.



**Disclaimer:** The statements, opinions and data contained in this publication are solely those of the individual authors and contributors and not of the publisher and the editor(s). The appearance of advertisements in the journal is not a warranty, endorsement, or approval of the products or services advertised or of their effectiveness, quality or safety. The publisher and the editor(s) disclaim responsibility for any injury to persons or property resulting form any ideas, methods, instructions or products referred to in the content or advertisements.

**Subscription Rates:** Subscriptions run for a full calendar year.
Prices are given per year.

| | |
|---|---|
| **Print:** | EUR 203.00 + postage and handling |
| **Online:** | EUR 203.00 |
| **Combined** (print+online): | EUR 253.00 + postage and handling |

**Postage and handling** (added to print and print+online):
EUR 16.00 (Germany), EUR 25.00 (Rest of World)

**Discount subscription prices:**
Please enquire about reduced rates for members of related societies.

**Back Volumes and Single Issues:** Information on availability and prices of single print issues and print or electronic back volumes can be obtained from Customer Service at aboservice@karger.com

**For customers in Germany:** Please contact your local bookstore or
S. Karger Verlag für Medizin und Naturwissenschaften GmbH
Wilhelmstr. 20A, 79098 Freiburg (Germany)
Tel. +49 761 45 20 70, Fax +49 761 45 20 714
aboservice@karger.com

**For customers in all other countries:** Please contact your bookshop or
S. Karger AG
Allschwilerstr. 10, 4009 Basel (Switzerland)
Tel. +41 61 3 06 11 11, Fax +41 61 3 06 12 34
karger@karger.com

**Advertising:** Correspondence should be addressed to the publisher.
S. Karger Verlag für Medizin und Naturwissenschaften GmbH
Attn. Ellen Zimmermann (Head of Marketing)
e.zimmermann@karger.com
Price list No. 24 of January 1, 2017 is effective.

**Publisher:** S. Karger Verlag für Medizin und Naturwissenschaften GmbH
Wilhelmstr. 20A, 79098 Freiburg (Germany)
www.karger.de, information@karger.com

**V.i.S.d.P.** (Person responsible according to the German Press Law):
Sibylle Gross

**Type setting and printing:** Kraft Premium GmbH, 76275 Ettlingen, Germany.
Printed on acid-free and non-aging paper (ISO 9706).

ISBN 978-3-318-06008-9
e-ISBN 978-3-318-06009-6

**Indexing/Abstracting**
Listed in bibliographic services, including:
PubMed / PubMed Central / Web of Science / Emerging Sources Citation Index / Google Scholar / Scopus / Embase / Pathway Studio / WorldCat

Visceral Medicine

Review Article

Visc Med 2017;33:435–441
DOI: 10.1159/000480100

Published online: December 4, 2017

# A Comparison of Pitfalls after ALPPS Stage 1 or Portal Vein Embolization in Small-for-Size Setting Hepatectomies

Andreas A. Schnitzbauer

Clinic for General and Visceral Surgery, University Hospital Frankfurt, Goethe-University Frankfurt/Main, Frankfurt/M., Germany

**Keywords**

ALPPS · Portal vein embolization, PVE · Liver resection · Small-for-size setting · Pre-completion pitfalls · Failure

**Summary**

**Background:** Portal vein embolization (PVE) followed by resection and associating liver partition and portal vein ligation for staged hepatectomy (ALPPS) are tools to enable liver resections in small-for-size settings. **Methods:** A systematic review of the literature and comparison of pitfalls between PVE and resection and after ALPPS stage 1 were performed. **Results:** Evidence levels were as low as 4 for both procedures. 20 publications were identified with reports on post-PVE or post-ALPPS stage 1 pitfalls. A total of 2,758 patients treated with PVE followed by resection and 698 patients undergoing ALPPS were analyzed. Pitfalls identified were failure to advance to resection (PVE: high (20%)/ALPPS: low (1%); p = 0.0001), tumor progression (PVE: high/ALPPS: low); insufficient hypertrophy (PVE: frequent/ALPPS: rare), and inter-stage liver failure (PVE: rare/ALPPS: frequent). However, in-house mortality was still very high after ALPPS (7 vs. 3%, p = 0.0001) in a pooled analysis. **Conclusion:** PVE is a well-established technique to induce hypertrophy in small-for-size settings. The weakness of PVE is that it may fail to advance to resection. Inter-stage liver failure in ALPPS triggers post-stage 2 mortality. Prolongation of the inter-stage interval to overcome liver failure or cancellation of the resection stage combined with adherence to defined indications has the potential to make ALPPS much safer and decrease mortality rates. Level of evidence is low for both techniques.



## Introduction

Portal vein embolization (PVE) was first described by Kinoshita et al. [1] and Makuuchi et al. [2] more than 30 years ago. Its establishment in modern liver surgery allowed surgeons to perform safe resections in small-for-size settings (surgically possible but functionally not) where the future liver remnant (FLR) increases in size in response to PVE and the patient does not show signs of disease progression. With the interventional embolization or surgical ligation of the portal vein, the FLR is stimulated, obtaining growth rates of 25–50% within 4–6 weeks [3]. In a second step, the tumor may be resected safely without driving patients into fatal post-hepatectomy liver failure, especially after extensive pre-resection chemotherapy [4, 5]. Until recently, PVE was an absolute sovereign and a monopolist with regard to enlarging the FLR. However, only 5 years ago, the group of Hans Schlitt established a new technique of 2-stage hepatectomy to induce FLR growth. The new technique combined portal vein ligation and parenchymal transection during the first stage of surgery, a short interval for FLR growth and regeneration (10 days), and the removal of tumor-bearing liver in the second step of surgery. The kinetic growth rates of the FLR were around 75% within 8–12 days after stage 1 surgery and were larger than any other report so far [6, 7]. Clavien and de Santibañes [8] established a now commonly used descriptive name for this new procedure: associating liver partition and portal vein ligation for staged hepatectomy, the so-called ALPPS procedure. However, just as most innovations suffer from initial throwbacks, the exploration phase of ALPPS also unveiled relevant morbidity in patients as well as unacceptable high mortality rates, especially in unselected patient cohorts and in certain indications such as perihilar cholangiocarcinoma [9–11]. Driven by the ALPPS registry, certain recommendations have been made concerning indications, surgical-technical modifications, and patient management, discussed and worded during the 1st international ALPPS consensus meeting in

KARGER

Fax +49 761 4 52 07 14
Information@Karger.com
www.karger.com



Accessible online at:
www.karger.com/vis

Prof. Andreas A. Schnitzbauer, MD, FACS, FEBS
Clinic for General and Visceral Surgery
University Hospital Frankfurt, Goethe University Frankfurt/Main
Theodor-Stern-Kai 7, 60590 Frankfurt, Germany
andreas.schnitzbauer@kgu.de

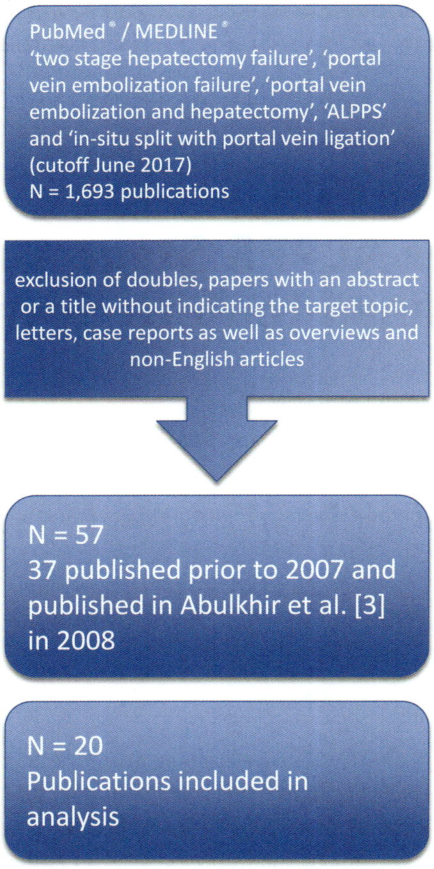


**Fig. 1.** Flow chart of paper selection.

Hamburg in 2015 [12]. Nonetheless, the evidence level for ALPPS benefit is still low, with no prospective randomized controlled trials comparing PVE and ALPPS so far. Besides, blinded by the 100% feasibility rate and the tremendous rates of hypertrophy, almost nobody focused on what happened between stages 1 and 2 of ALPPS. This time period, in which the critical pathophysiological damage occurs, is very likely to determine the further course of patients after ALPPS stage 2. Therefore, a systematic review was performed to detect and compare the pitfalls occurring in the interval between PVE and subsequent resection and between ALPPS stage 1 and 2.

## Methods

A PubMed/MEDLINE search was performed for the search terms '2-stage hepatectomy failure', 'portal vein embolization failure', 'portal vein embolization and hepatectomy', 'ALPPS', and 'in-situ split with portal vein ligation'. Doubles and non-suitable articles were excluded. The search was performed 2 times to minimize the risk of selection bias. Articles were included in the analysis when the abstract reported failure rates, complications, or pitfalls after PVE or ALPPS stage 1. In more detail, target information was extracted focusing on inter-stage pitfalls that predicted liver failure after stage 2 in ALPPS, and post-PVE factors hindering progress to subsequent resection. Failure in PVE was defined as an event that did not allow advancement to resection, and in the ALPPS procedure, as critical factors that occurred between stages 1 and 2, discouraging advancement to stage 2. Data were presented in a descriptive manner using total numbers, proportions, and risk factors where available. A cumulative pooled outcome analysis of patients was performed to analyze failure rate and in-house mortality. Evidence levels for benefit in both PVE and ALPPS were determined using the latest Oxford Centre of Evidence-Based Medicine recommendations [13]. Statistical analyses were performed with Review Manager (RevMan) Version 5.2. (The Nordic Cochrane Centre, The Cochrane Collaboration, Copenhagen, 2012).

## Results

*Number of Publications and Selection*

A total of 1,693 publications were detected with the search terms described above until the cut-off date of June 2017. After exclusion of doubles, papers with an abstract or title not indicating the target topic, letters, case reports, as well as overviews and non-English articles, 57 papers remained. Of those, 37 were published before the year 2007 and were in large part analyzed in the meta-analysis by Abulkhir et al. in 2008 [3]. A total of 20 papers remained for analysis to compare ALPPS and PVE, focusing on pitfalls leading to failure of the intended treatment completion. Figure 1 displays a flowchart of the paper selection.

*Evidence Levels for the Publications Analyzed*

Evidence levels were generally low for the interventions dealt with in this review (PVE followed by resection or ALPPS). Of the 20 publications analyzed, 2 were systematic reviews of case series and case-control studies comparing the 2 techniques, 13 were case series, and 5 were case-control studies. There were no cohort studies. This accounted for an overall evidence level of 4 for both PVE and ALPPS, as the review by Abulkhir et al. [3] was not a meta-analysis of randomized controlled trials.

*General Observations*

Resection strategies using PVE or ALPPS are infrequently employed at a rate of approximately 8 times per year (range 3.2–15.6) in very selected high-volume hepatobiliary centers. Unfortunately, most centers do not provide the whole volume of their liver program. Therefore, the proportion of liver resections in small-for-size settings using ALPPS or PVE remains an educated guess. Nonetheless, the total numbers given above are likely to be representative.

*Pooled Outcome Analysis of Failure and In-House Mortality Comparing ALPPS versus PVE Followed by Resection*

Strikingly, the failure rate of PVE was considerably higher than that of ALPPS (fig. 2). A total number of 555 patients could not be resected after PVE whereas 1,956 were resected. In comparison, only 8 patients did not proceed to ALPPS stage 2, while 726 patients completed the treatment successfully. The difference was highly significant ($p = 0.0001$). However, the in-house mortality

| Study or Subgroup | ALPPS Events | ALPPS Total | PVE and resection Events | PVE and resection Total | Weight | Odds Ratio M-H, Random, 95% CI |
|---|---|---|---|---|---|---|
| pooled data | 8 | 734 | 555 | 2511 | 100.0% | 0.04 [0.02, 0.08] |
| **Total (95% CI)** | | **734** | | **2511** | **100.0%** | **0.04 [0.02, 0.08]** |
| Total events | 8 | | 555 | | | |

Heterogeneity: Not applicable
Test for overall effect: Z = 9.06 (P < 0.00001)

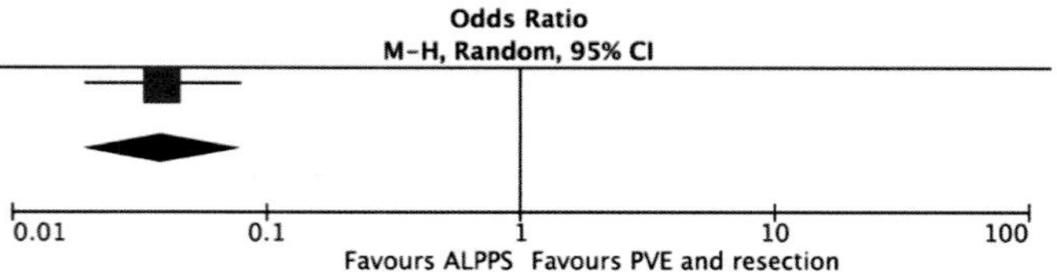


**Fig. 2.** Forrest plot of failure to progress to resection – ALPPS procedure compared to PVE followed by resection.

| Study or Subgroup | ALPPS Events | ALPPS Total | PVE and resection Events | PVE and resection Total | Weight | Odds Ratio M-H, Random, 95% CI |
|---|---|---|---|---|---|---|
| pooled data | 60 | 717 | 75 | 2348 | 100.0% | 2.77 [1.95, 3.93] |
| **Total (95% CI)** | | **717** | | **2348** | **100.0%** | **2.77 [1.95, 3.93]** |
| Total events | 60 | | 75 | | | |

Heterogeneity: Not applicable
Test for overall effect: Z = 5.69 (P < 0.00001)

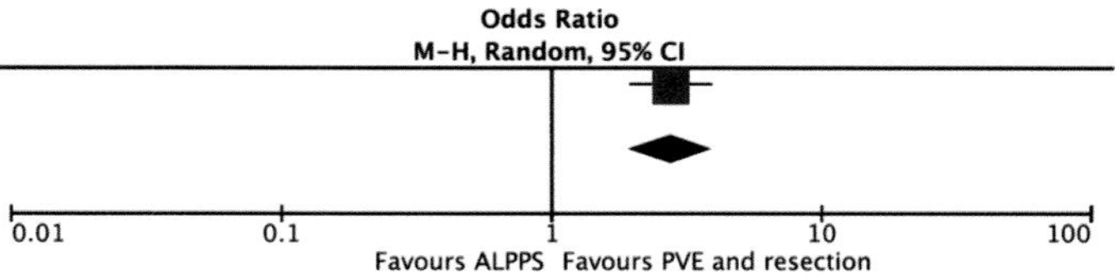


**Fig. 3.** Forrest plot of in-house mortality – ALPPS procedure compared to PVE followed by resection.

after PVE was significantly lower than that after ALPPS (fig. 3). Here, we see a completely different picture. After PVE and resection, only 75 patients died and 2,273 survived. In contrast, after the ALPPS procedure, 60 patients died compared to 657 survivors. This difference was again highly significant (p = 0.0001).

*Pitfalls Detected after PVE Hindering the Advancement to Resection*

In the systematic review by Abulkhir et al. [3], the overall morbidity after PVE (including post-resection complications) was very low with 2.2% of all cases. Insufficient hypertrophy after PVE and disease progression were the most frequent reasons why resection was not performed. Besides, other authors described a worsening of comorbidities during the waiting time after PVE and a misinterpretation of resectability as additional factors. However, there were also factors directly related to PVE; nausea/pain, thrombosis in the mesenterico-portal veins, esophageal varicose bleeding, liver hematoma, and incomplete or wrong embolization were serious albeit rare PVE complications that could be hazardous for the patients.

*Pitfalls Detected after ALPPS Stage 1 That Led to Adverse Outcome after Stage 2*

Descriptions of inter-stage pitfalls after ALPPS remain rare. Truant et al. [14] performed the first systematic analysis. The authors described that the failure rate after ALPPS was 5% due to insufficient growth, portal vein thrombosis, and inter-stage death, and that a delay in the planned procedure beyond day 9 was seen in more than 50% of patients. Schadde et al. [15] described that inter-stage liver failure and an inter-stage MELD score >10 were highly predictive for mortality after stage 2. In detail, 21 of 28 patients with liver failure after stage 1 died within 90 days after stage 2, especially in the case of a MELD score >10 (odds ratio 3.9–4.9). Surgery-related fatal liver failure was finally confirmed in the publication by Linecker et al. [16]. Extracted data for all analyzed publications are displayed in table 1. Table 2 summarizes the findings described above.

## Discussion

The technique of PVE followed by resection was developed over several decades and is a well-established tool in small-for-size settings in liver surgery [1]. ALPPS, in contrast, is the new kid on the block. It was published only 5 years ago, and the first procedure was performed 10 years ago [6]. PVE followed by resection was developed within a considerable timeframe without competition from any other procedure, and was properly assessed. That way, data from long-term studies were obtained. ALPPS revealed certain flaws in its beginning but was developed properly by the introduction of a registry which made the procedure safer. Nonetheless, this review showed that pre-resection pitfalls remain poorly reported in both PVE and ALPPS, and that the evidence level is low with publications of predominantly level 4 [13]. Strikingly, the failure to advance to liver resection was rather high in patients with PVE. The reasons for PVE failure are well analyzed and consistently described throughout the literature; however, they still contribute to a failure rate of approximately 20% of all procedures. Reports on ALPPS failure after the stage 1 operation are still very rare. Manuscripts focusing on reasons for failure after ALPPS have so far only been published by Truant et al. [14], Schadde et al. [15], and Linecker et al. [16]. ALPPS still results in a very high in-house mortality and thus also impairs the oncologic outcome of the patients; however, mortality has somewhat improved with better patient selection along with the adherence to the recommended avoidance of certain indications such as perihilar cholangiocarcinoma [11, 17].

In this review, the overall mortality for the ALPPS procedure was 7% compared to 3% after PVE followed by liver resection. This demonstrates that the implementation of correct indications for ALPPS is pivotal. Additionally, we learn that inter-stage complications must lead to a reconsideration of whether to delay or even stop the progression to stage 2. Since 21 of 28 patients with inter-stage liver failure died after completion of stage 2, manifestation of liver failure (International Study Group of Liver Surgery [4]) after stage 1 should be regarded as a contraindication for completing

**Tab. 1.** Overview of studies and extracted data from the literature

| Author [ref.] | Journal | City | Year | Evidence level | Number of patients over time, n | Failure rate, % (n) | Reasons for failure and complications | Modality |
|---|---|---|---|---|---|---|---|---|
| Abulkhir [3] | Ann Surg | London | 2008 | review of case series and case-control studies | 1,088 | 15 | 2.2% overall morbidity of PVE<br>insufficient hypertrophy and progress as most frequent reasons for failure | PVE in mixed indications prior to major liver resection |
| Tsai [20] | HPB (Oxford) | Baltimore | 2010 | case series | 45 in 14 years | 22 (10) | progress (n = 7)<br>poor ECOG status (n = 1)<br>death before resection (n = 2) | PVE + CTx in CRLM |
| Massimino [21] | HPB (Oxford) | Portland | 2012 | case series | 23 in 5 years | 13 (3) | PVE complications (n = 7)<br>pain/nausea (n = 2)<br>SMV thrombosis (n = 1)<br>liver hematoma (n = 1)<br>wrong target vein (n = 2) | PVE in CRLM |
| Lam [22] | HPB (Oxford) | Sydney | 2013 | systematic review of case series and case-control studies | 459 | 23 (107) | progress (n = 94)<br>insufficient hypertrophy (n = 4)<br>PVT (n = 4)<br>death before resection (n = 2) | PVE + CTx+/ablation (classic TSH concepts) in CRLM |
| Shindoh [23] | J Am Coll Surg | Houston | 2013 | case series | 141 | 27.8 (40) | progress (n = 27)<br>insufficient regeneration (n = 5)<br>comorbidities (n = 8)<br>incomplete embolization (n = 3)<br>PVE complications (n = 2) | PVE in CRLM |
| Shindoh [18] | Br J Surg | Houston | 2013 | case-control study | 265<br>139 PVE/<br>126 primary resection | 37 (51) in PVE | progress<br>insufficient hypertrophy<br>tumor load during laparotomy | PVE vs. conventional primary surgery in CRLM |
| Schadde [24] | HPB (Oxford) | Zurich | 2013 | case-control study | 35 TSH vs.<br>163 conventional resections in 9 years | 0% failure, only 9/35 with PVE | N.A. | N.A. |
| Schadde [17] | Ann Surg | Zurich | 2014 | case series | 202 | 0 | no analysis of inter-stage risk factors<br>RBCT, OR time > 300 min.,<br>age > 60 years, and non-CRLM indication were risk factors of adverse outcome | ALPPS in mixed indications |
| Leung [25] | J Am Coll Surg | New York | 2014 | case series | 153 in 13 years | N.A. | degree of hypertrophy and growth rate of <2.66% of total liver volume/week were predictive for liver failure after resection | PVE in CRLM |

**Table 1.** *Continued on next page*

**Table 1.** *Continued*

| Author [ref.] | Journal | City | Year | Evidence level | Number of patients over time, n | Failure rate, % (n) | Reasons for failure and complications | Modality |
|---|---|---|---|---|---|---|---|---|
| Shindoh [26] | J Gastrointest Surg | Houston | 2014 | case series | 358 in 23 years | 33 (118) without curative approach | progress (n = 19)<br>irresectable (n = 25)<br>insufficient regeneration (n = 13)<br>comorbidities (n = 19)<br>PVT (n = 8)<br>PVE complications (n = 3)<br>hematoma (n = 2)<br>esophageal bleeding (n = 1) | PVE in mixed indications |
| Truant [14] | Eur J Surg Oncol | Lille | 2015 | case series | 62 | 5 (3) | insufficient hypertrophy (n = 1)<br>PVT (n = 1)<br>death (n = 1)<br>delayed > 9 d (n = 32) | ALPPS mixed indications |
| Schadde [15] | Ann Surg | Zurich | 2015 | case series | 320 | 1.6 (5) | liver failure after stage 1 (ISGLS)<br>MELD > 10<br>(risk factors for mortality after stage 2) | ALPPS in CRLM |
| Hernandez-Alejandro [27] | Surgery | London-Ontario | 2015 | case series | 14 in 2 years | 0 | no complications reported | ALPPS in CRLM |
| Ratti [28] | Ann Surg Onc | Milan | 2015 | case-control study | 48<br>36 TSH/12 ALPPS | 6 (2) in TSH<br>0 in ALPPS | disease progression (n = 2) | TSH with PVE and ALPPS |
| Passot [29] | J Am Coll Surg | Houston | 2016 | case series | 109 in 12 years | 18 (20) | progress (n = 12)<br>insufficient hypertrophy (n = 5)<br>PVE-complications (n = 3) | PVE in CRLM |
| Sparrelid [30] | Langenbecks Arch Surg | Stockholm | 2016 | case series | 11 | 100 | insufficient hypertrophy following PVE | rescue ALPPS |
| De Santibañes [31] | Langenbecks Arch Surg | Buenos Aires | 2016 | case series | 4 | 0 | N.A. | ALPPS with PVE, no-touch anterior approach, partial parenchymal transection in mixed indications |
| Adam [32] | Br J Surg | Paris | 2016 | case-control study | 58<br>41 TSH/17 ALPPS | 36 (15) in TSH,<br>0 in ALPPS | similar complication rate but worse overall outcome in ALPPS | ALPPS vs. TSH with PVE in CRLM |
| Cieslak [33] | Surgery | Amsterdam | 2017 | case series | 63 | 40 (18) | liver failure after surgery (3 fatal)<br>insufficient hypertrophy (n = 4)<br>surgery technically not feasible (n = 1)<br>death before resection (n = 1) | PVE in CRLM |
| Linecker [16] | Surgery | Zurich | 2017 | case-control study | 67<br>22 partial/22 matched/<br>23 historic | 0 | surgery-related fatal liver failure grade C after stage 2 (n = 2) | ALPPS partial vs. full in CRLM |

PVE = Portal vein embolization; ALPPS = associating liver partition and portal vein ligation for staged hepatectomy; CTx = chemotherapy; CRLM = colorectal liver metastases; SMV = superior mesenteric vein; PVT = portal vein thrombosis; TSH = 2-stage hepatectomy; N.A. = not available; RBCT = red blood cell transfusion; OT = operating time; ISGLS = International Study Group of Liver Surgery.

**Tab. 2.** Summary of key findings

| | PVE and resection | ALPPS | Conclusion/recommendations |
|---|---|---|---|
| Technique used, n (over years) | >30 | >10 | ALPPS data still in phase of exploration (2b); however, recommendations indicate entry into assessment phase (3) of surgical innovations [34] |
| Evidence level | level 4 (low) | level 4 (low) | no randomized controlled trials, no direct comparison of the 2 techniques available |
| In-house mortality | acceptable | still too high | favoring PVE |
| Time interval before final resection | 2–4 weeks | 7–15 days | favoring ALPPS; however, time interval can be valuable for identifying patients that do not profit from progressing to final procedure for tumor biological reasons patients with ALPPS inter-stage complications may profit from a longer interval between stages |
| Failure rate (no progression to final resection) | very high | very low | favoring ALPPS |
| Progress | frequent | rare | may be a selection criterion and thus prevent postsurgical in-house mortality; OS of intention-to-treat analysis for PVE unclear |
| PVE complications | rare | N.A. | PVE = established procedure |
| Insufficient hypertrophy | frequent | rare | favoring ALPPS, especially as rescue ALPPS after failed PVE |
| Inter-stage liver failure | rare | frequent | favoring PVE; may lead to delay of ALPPS stage 2 making it a safer procedure |
| Inter-stage death | rare | rare | not a common problem |

PVE = Portal vein embolization; ALPPS = associating liver partition and portal vein ligation for staged hepatectomy; OS = overall survival; N.A. = not available.

ALPPS as outlined by Schadde et al. [15]. The stage 2 operation can either be cancelled or be performed only in the case of recovery from liver failure. This has 2 advantages: First, the rate of liver failure-associated mortality would be reduced, and second, although potentially conflicting with the rapid hypertrophy principle of ALPPS, a longer waiting time could improve biologic selection. If the failure to advance to stage 2 increased from the currently reported rate of 1% to 5 or even 10%, and if mortality rates were at the same time reduced to 3%, ALPPS would have the potential be a more successful procedure than PVE. The overall number of patients with ALPPS failure would be much lower than that of those with PVE failure, resulting in better overall survival in an intention-to-treat setting due to the lower proportion of palliative treatment compared to patients with failure after PVE [18, 19].

The limitations of this analysis lie in the low level of evidence for both procedures. Double-checking all the included publications minimized the selection bias. However, the fact that only retrospective case series exist and the lack of head-to-head randomized controlled trials allowed only a descriptive comparison.

In conclusion, PVE is still the best option enabling safe liver resection in small-for-size settings. The pre-resection pitfalls after PVE are well described; however, failure to advance to liver resection after PVE leads 20% of patients to palliative treatment, resulting in a dramatic decrease in long-term oncologic survival. In patients with liver resection after PVE, however, the prognosis is still outstanding in this medically complex patient group. The outline of indications for ALPPS has much improved, but inter-stage problems are still poorly described. When inter-stage liver failure is avoided, the long-term prognosis after the ALPPS procedure is good. Either prolonging the inter-stage phase or cancelling the stage 2 procedure may allow the prevention of perioperative deaths in ALPPS, including an oncologically sound biologic selection.

## Disclosure Statement

There are no conflicts of interest.

## References


1 Kinoshita H, Sakai K, Hirohashi K, et al: Preoperative portal vein embolization for hepatocellular carcinoma. World J Surg 1986;10:803–808.

2 Makuuchi M, Thai BL, Takayasu K, et al: Preoperative portal embolization to increase safety of major hepatectomy for hilar bile duct carcinoma: a preliminary report. Surgery 1990;107:521–527.

3 Abulkhir A, Limongelli P, Healey AJ, et al: Preoperative portal vein embolization for major liver resection: a meta-analysis. Ann Surg 2008;247:49–57.

4 Rahbari NN, Garden OJ, Padbury R, et al: Posthepatectomy liver failure: a definition and grading by the International Study Group of Liver Surgery (ISGLS). Surgery 2011;149:713–724.
5 Vauthey J-N, Pawlik TM, Ribero D, et al: Chemotherapy regimen predicts steatohepatitis and an increase in 90-day mortality after surgery for hepatic colorectal metastases. J Clin Oncol 2006;24:2065–2072.
6 Schnitzbauer AA, Lang SA, Goessmann H, et al: Right portal vein ligation combined with in situ splitting induces rapid left lateral liver lobe hypertrophy enabling 2-staged extended right hepatic resection in small-for-size settings. Ann Surg 2012;255:405–414.
7 Schadde E, Schnitzbauer AA, Tschuor C, et al: Systematic review and meta-analysis of feasibility, safety, and efficacy of a novel procedure: associating liver partition and portal vein ligation for staged hepatectomy. Ann Surg Oncol 2015;22:3109–3120.
8 De Santibañes E, Clavien P-A: Playing Play-Doh to prevent postoperative liver failure: the 'ALPPS' approach. Ann Surg 2012;255:415–417.
9 Oldhafer KJ, Donati M, Jenner RM, et al: ALPPS for patients with colorectal liver metastases: effective liver hypertrophy, but early tumor recurrence. World J Surg 2014;38:1504–1509.
10 Nadalin S, Capobianco I, Li J, et al: Indications and limits for associating liver partition and portal vein ligation for staged hepatectomy (ALPPS). Lessons learned from 15 cases at a single centre. Z Gastroenterol 2014;52:35–42.
11 Olthof PB, Coelen RJS, Wiggers JK, et al: High mortality after ALPPS for perihilar cholangiocarcinoma: case-control analysis including the first series from the international ALPPS registry. HPB (Oxford) 2017;19:381–387.
12 Oldhafer KJ, Stavrou GA, van Gulik TM, et al: ALPPS – where do we stand, where do we go?: eight recommendations from the first international expert meeting. Ann Surg 2016;263:839–841.
13 Howick J, Chalmers I, Glasziou P, et al: The 2011 Oxford CEBM Levels of Evidence: Introductory Document. Oxford Centre for Evidence-Based Medicine, *www.cebm.net/index.aspx?o=5653*.
14 Truant S, Scatton O, Dokmak S, et al: Associating liver partition and portal vein ligation for staged hepatectomy (ALPPS): impact of the inter-stages course on morbi-mortality and implications for management. Eur J Surg Oncol 2015;41:674–682.
15 Schadde E, Raptis DA, Schnitzbauer AA, et al: Prediction of mortality after ALPPS stage-1: an analysis of 320 patients from the International ALPPS Registry. Ann Surg 2015;262:780–786.
16 Linecker M, Kambakamba P, Reiner CS, et al: How much liver needs to be transected in ALPPS? A translational study investigating the concept of less invasiveness. Surgery 2017;161:453–464.
17 Schadde E, Ardiles V, Robles-Campos R, et al: Early survival and safety of ALPPS: first report of the International ALPPS Registry. Ann Surg 2014;260:829–836, discussion 836–838.
18 Shindoh J, Tzeng C-WD, Aloia TA, et al: Portal vein embolization improves rate of resection of extensive colorectal liver metastases without worsening survival. Br J Surg 2013;100:1777–1783.
19 Folprecht G, Gruenberger T, Bechstein WO, et al: Tumour response and secondary resectability of colorectal liver metastases following neoadjuvant chemotherapy with cetuximab: the CELIM randomised phase 2 trial. Lancet Oncol 2010;11:38–47.
20 Tsai S, Marques HP, de Jong MC, et al: Two-stage strategy for patients with extensive bilateral colorectal liver metastases. HPB (Oxford) 2010;12:262–269.
21 Massimino KP, Kolbeck KJ, Enestvedt CK, et al: Safety and efficacy of preoperative right portal vein embolization in patients at risk for postoperative liver failure following major right hepatectomy. HPB (Oxford) 2012;14:14–19.
22 Lam VWT, Laurence JM, Johnston E, et al: A systematic review of two-stage hepatectomy in patients with initially unresectable colorectal liver metastases. HPB (Oxford) 2013;15:483–491.
23 Shindoh J, Vauthey J-N, Zimmitti G, et al: Analysis of the efficacy of portal vein embolization for patients with extensive liver malignancy and very low future liver remnant volume, including a comparison with the associating liver partition with portal vein ligation for staged hepatectomy approach. J Am Coll Surg 2013;217:126–133, discussion 133–134.
24 Schadde E, Slankamenac K, Breitenstein S, et al: Are two-stage hepatectomies associated with more complications than one-stage procedures? HPB (Oxford) 2013;15:411–417.
25 Leung U, Simpson AL, Araujo RLC, et al: Remnant growth rate after portal vein embolization is a good early predictor of post-hepatectomy liver failure. J Am Coll Surg 2014;219:620–630.
26 Shindoh J, Tzeng C-WD, Aloia TA, et al: Safety and efficacy of portal vein embolization before planned major or extended hepatectomy: an institutional experience of 358 patients. J Gastrointest Surg 2014;18:45–51.
27 Hernandez-Alejandro R, Bertens KA, Pineda-Solis K, et al: Can we improve the morbidity and mortality associated with the associating liver partition with portal vein ligation for staged hepatectomy (ALPPS) procedure in the management of colorectal liver metastases? Surgery 2015;157:194–201.
28 Ratti F, Schadde E, Masetti M, et al: Strategies to increase the resectability of patients with colorectal liver metastases: a multi-center case-match analysis of ALPPS and conventional two-stage hepatectomy. Ann Surg Oncol 2015;22:1933–1942.
29 Passot G, Chun YS, Kopetz SE, et al: Predictors of safety and efficacy of 2-stage hepatectomy for bilateral colorectal liver metastases. J Am Coll Surg 2016;223:99–108.
30 Sparrelid E, Gilg S, Brismar TB, et al: Rescue ALPPS is efficient and safe after failed portal vein occlusion in patients with colorectal liver metastases. Langenbecks Arch Surg 2017;402:69–75.
31 De Santibañes E, Alvarez FA, Ardiles V, et al: Inverting the ALPPS paradigm by minimizing first stage impact: the Mini-ALPPS technique. Langenbecks Arch Surg 2016;401:557–563.
32 Adam R, Imai K, Castro Benitez C, et al: Outcome after associating liver partition and portal vein ligation for staged hepatectomy and conventional two-stage hepatectomy for colorectal liver metastases. Br J Surg 2016;103:1521–1529.
33 Cieslak KP, Huisman F, Bais T, et al: Future remnant liver function as predictive factor for the hypertrophy response after portal vein embolization. Surgery 2017;162:37–47.
34 McCulloch P, Altman DG, Campbell WB, et al: No surgical innovation without evaluation: the IDEAL recommendations. Lancet 2009;374:1105–1112.

Visceral Medicine

**Review Article**

Visc Med 2017;33:442–448
DOI: 10.1159/000480385

Published online: November 30, 2017

# Current Modalities for the Assessment of Future Remnant Liver Function

Fadi Rassam[a] Pim B. Olthof[a] Roelof J. Bennink[b] Thomas M. van Gulik[a]

[a] Department of Surgery, Academic Medical Center, Amsterdam, The Netherlands;
[b] Department of Radiology and Nuclear Medicine, Academic Medical Center, Amsterdam, The Netherlands

**Keywords**
Liver function tests · Liver resection · Posthepatectomy liver failure

**Summary**
While imaging studies such as computed tomography or magnetic resonance imaging allow the volumetric assessment of the liver segments, only indirect information is provided concerning the quality of the liver parenchyma and its actual functional capacity. Assessment of liver function is therefore crucial in the preoperative workup of patients who require extensive liver resection and in whom portal vein embolization is considered. This review deals with the modalities currently available for the measurement of liver function. Passive liver function tests include biochemical parameters and clinical grading systems such as the Child-Pugh and MELD scores. Dynamic quantitative tests of liver function can be based on clearance capacity tests such as the indocyanine green (ICG) clearance test. Although widely used, discrepancies have been reported for the ICG clearance test in relation with clinical outcome. Nuclear imaging studies have the advantage of providing simultaneous morphologic (visual) and physiologic (quantitative functional) information about the liver. In addition, regional (segmental) differentiation allows specific functional assessment of the future remnant liver. Technetium-99m ($^{99m}$Tc)-galactosyl human serum albumin scintigraphy and $^{99m}$Tc-mebrofenin hepatobiliary scintigraphy potentially identify patients at risk for post-resectional liver failure who might benefit from liver-augmenting techniques. As there is no one test that can measure all the components of liver function, liver functional reserve is estimated based on a combination of clinical parameters and quantitative liver function tests.



## Introduction

Liver-augmenting techniques such as portal vein embolization (PVE), 2-stage resection, and ALPPS (associating liver partition and portal vein ligation for staged hepatectomy) have pushed forward the frontiers of liver resection, resulting in an increase in the number of patients eligible for major liver resection. Judicious use of these modalities now offers patients with extensive tumor load, complex tumors, or highly compromised livers a chance for a curative resection. This aggressive surgical approach, however, comes with substantial morbidity and a mortality higher than accepted with standard resections.

The most dramatic complication after liver resection is the occurrence of posthepatectomy liver failure (PHLF) with reported mortality rates of up to 80% [1]. Management of PHLF is largely supportive, while these patients seldom are candidates for salvage (cadaveric) liver transplantation as the tumor burden underlying these extensive resections usually by far exceeds accepted criteria for liver replacement. Resection in these patients therefore remains a challenge and requires special skills and experience on the part of the hepatobiliary surgeons and all specialties involved in the preoperative assessment.

Many efforts have been directed toward predicting liver functional reserve preoperatively, taking into account the extent of resection considered necessary to remove all tumor and the quality of the liver parenchyma. We usually rely on computed tomography (CT) volumetric studies for the assessment of patients requiring major liver resection; however, while many of the patients referred for resection have undergone extensive chemotherapy with resulting steatotic or microvascular changes to their livers, the volume of the future remnant liver (FRL) may not correlate with the function of the FRL [2–4].

In this overview, we describe the current modalities available for the assessment of the FRL in patients scheduled for major hepatic resection. In patients with small-for-size FRL or insufficient FRL function, who are exposed to liver-augmenting techniques, we also

KARGER

Fax +49 761 4 52 07 14
Information@Karger.com
www.karger.com



Accessible online at:
www.karger.com/vis

Thomas M. van Gulik, MD
Department of Surgery (IA1-119)
Academic Medical Center
Meibergdreef 9, 1105 AZ Amsterdam, The Netherlands
t.m.vangulik@amc.nl

discuss the use of these functional tests to monitor the hypertrophy response of the FRL.

## Passive Liver Function Tests

*Biochemical Parameters*

Passive liver function tests include biochemical parameters and clinical grading systems. The term 'liver function tests' to indicate a set of conventional plasma parameters is confusing because they do not represent the functional components of the liver except for clotting factors which are synthesized by the liver. The aminotransaminase enzymes, aspartate transferase (AST) and alanine transferase (ALT), are markers of liver damage and correlate with the extent of hepatocellular necrosis [5]. Although a persisting release of these enzymes will ultimately result in the loss of liver functional capacity, they are not parameters of function per se. Albumin and clotting factors, however, are exclusively synthesized by the liver and their plasma concentrations are therefore used as indirect indicators of liver function. The plasma bilirubin concentration provides indirect information on the uptake, conjugation, and excretion function of the liver. However, plasma bilirubin levels are also influenced by extrahepatic factors such as increased production of bilirubin or bile duct obstruction [6, 7].

Hyaluronic acid (HA), a more recent biochemical parameter, is a glycosaminoglycan which is produced by connective tissue cells and synovial cells and is exclusively taken up from the blood and metabolized by the sinusoidal endothelial cells of the liver. HA concentration in the blood may therefore be considered a functional test of the liver sinusoidal endothelial cells and as such of the whole liver. In a series of patients with primary and secondary liver tumors, we found a significant positive correlation between HA and almost every conventional liver parameter. A significant correlation was demonstrated between plasma concentrations of HA and the indocyanine green (ICG) retention test in which ICG retention of 15% corresponded with a HA level of 233 ng/ml (normal plasma HA values: 0–75 ng/ml) (unpublished results). A similar correlation between plasma HA and ICG retention rate at 15 min (ICG-R15) was reported by Nanashima et al. [8].

*Clinical Grading Systems*

Clinical grading systems combine several biochemical parameters together with clinical symptoms of insufficient liver function. The Child-Pugh score is a widely used clinical scoring systems which includes total bilirubin plasma level, albumin plasma level, and prothrombin time (PT) together with the presence or absence of encephalopathy and ascites. The Child-Pugh scoring system is particularly useful in selecting patients with hepatocellular carcinoma (HCC) and cirrhosis for resection or transplantation, as most class Child B and class Child C patients are candidates for transplantation, leaving class Child A patients for resection. In patients with liver metastases who usually have normal liver parenchyma and who are all classified as class Child A, the question then arises of how to identify those at risk of PHLF [9]. In these patients, the Child-Pugh score has been shown to be quite variable and may be unreliable for predicting the outcome of liver resections, especially in those with non-cirrhotic livers [10].

The MELD (Model for End-Stage Liver Disease) score was originally developed to predict short-term survival in patients undergoing transcutaneous intrahepatic portosystemic shunt procedures and has been adopted to stratify patients with end-stage liver disease awaiting transplantation. The MELD score includes serum bilirubin and creatinine levels and INR (International Normalized Ratio). MELD scores, however, did not predict morbidity or mortality after elective liver resection [11].

## Dynamic Quantitative Liver Function Tests

Biochemical liver function tests and clinical grading systems only provide indirect information about liver function. Therefore, especially in patients with non-cirrhotic livers, there is a need for objective tests to evaluate liver function in addition to clinical judgment. To this end, several dynamic quantitative tests of liver function have been devised [12]. As the various functional tests are based on different metabolic pathways, it is difficult to compare the value of each test in the context of risk assessment for liver resection. Several of these tests are discussed below.

*Indocyanine Green Clearance Test*

The ICG clearance test was initially devised for the measurement of blood flow, and later found clinical application in the assessment of liver function. It is now the most widely used quantitative liver function test. Although the test is routinely used in many Asian centers, its application has not been widely adopted in European centers. ICG is a tricarbocyanine dye that binds to albumin and is distributed uniformly in the blood within 2–3 min after intravenous injection. ICG is exclusively removed by the liver and excreted into the bile without intrahepatic conjugation [13]. Following administration, the blood level falls exponentially for about 20 min, by which time approximately 97% of the dye is excreted. ICG clearance is determined by serum sampling or pulse dye densitometry using an optical sensor placed on the finger [14, 15].

The ICG clearance test was found to be the best discriminating preoperative test for evaluating hepatic functional reserve in patients with HCC [16]. However, there are some drawbacks that may lead to discrepancies in relation to histological findings and clinical outcome. Discrepancies have been reported between ICG-R15 clearance rates and histological liver findings, and also clinical outcome [17]. Mortality has been noted in patients with normal ICG-R15, and survival in patients with poor outcome predicted on the basis of preoperative ICG-R15 [18]. One of the confounding factors in the measurement of ICG clearance is its flow dependency. Variation in hepatic blood flow such as that caused by intrahepatic shunting will influence the ICG clearance rate, rendering the test less predictive. Another point is that the ICG clearance test reflects the global liver function but does not take into account regional variations that may occur within the liver, obscuring a possible functional disadvantage of the segments to be preserved.

## Scintigraphic Liver Function Tests

Technetium-99m($^{99m}$Tc)-labeled diethylenetriaminepentaacetic acid (DTPA) galactosyl human serum albumin (GSA) scintigraphy and hepatobiliary scintigraphy (HBS) with $^{99m}$Tc-labeled iminodiacetic acid (IDA) derivatives are the most common representatives of this group [19]. Although both methods are based on different principles, both provide quantitative and visual information on total and regional hepatic function. $^{99m}$Tc-GSA scintigraphy is elaborated on and $^{99m}$Tc-mebrofenin HBS is discussed in this section.

*$^{99m}$Tc-GSA Scintigraphy*

The asialoglycoprotein receptor is specific for asialoglycoproteins which are formed after the removal of sialic acid from endogenous glycoproteins by sialidases. Asialoglycoproteins bind to asialoglycoprotein receptors on the hepatocyte sinusoidal surface and are subsequently taken up by receptor-mediated endocytosis and delivered to lysosomes for degradation. Chronic liver disease is associated with a decrease in the amount of asialoglycoprotein receptors and an accumulation of plasma asialoglycoproteins [20]. The $^{99m}$Tc-labeled asialoglycoprotein analog, $^{99m}$Tc-GSA, was clinically introduced as a new scintigraphy agent for imaging of the human hepatic receptor [21, 22]. $^{99m}$Tc-GSA is commercially available in an instant labelling kit in Japan.

The liver is the only uptake site for $^{99m}$Tc-GSA which makes it an ideal agent for liver function assessment. Furthermore, the uptake of $^{99m}$Tc-GSA is not affected by high bilirubin serum levels, making $^{99m}$Tc-GSA scintigraphy applicable even in cholestatic patients. Despite years of experience in South-East Asia, this radiopharmaceutical agent has not been released for clinical use in most European countries.

*Hepatobiliary Scintigraphy Using IDA Derivatives*

$^{99m}$Tc-IDA agents are lidocain analogs that are taken up by the hepatocytes and are directly excreted into the bile canaliculi without undergoing any biotransformation. $^{99m}$Tc-mebrofenin is the most hepatic-specific $^{99m}$Tc-IDA derivative [23]. Hepatic uptake of IDA agents via organic anion-transporting polypeptides (OATPs) can be influenced by high serum bilirubin levels as the same transporters are involved in the uptake of organic anions like bilirubin. Of all available IDA agents, $^{99m}$Tc-mebrofenin shows the lowest displacement by bilirubin in the case of hyperbilirubinemia [24]. The uptake, excretion, and lack of hepatic biotransformation of the IDA agents are similar to ICG. These properties make IDA agents suitable for the imaging of the hepatobiliary system and for use in the diagnosis of different biliary diseases [25]. The high hepatic uptake, low displacement by bilirubin, and, furthermore, low urinary excretion make mebrofenin the most suitable IDA agent for hepatic function assessment. We have used HBS in our center since the year 2000 for risk assessment of patients due to undergo any resection comprising three or more Couinaud segments [26, 27].

Camera-based measurement of the relative hepatic uptake rate was developed by Ekman et al. [28]. After intravenous injection of freshly prepared $^{99m}$Tc-mebrofenin, dynamic scintigraphy is performed with a dual-head gamma camera. Also here, the uptake of $^{99m}$Tc-mebrofenin is calculated by determining regions of interest (ROIs) around the heart, the liver, and the total field of view. Based on the ROIs, three time-activity curves can be generated. Using these parameters, it is possible to calculate the hepatic mebrofenin uptake ratio. Subsequently, a 3-dimensional single-photon emission computed tomography(SPECT)-CT is acquired during the time in which the tracer is accumulated in the liver. This provides quantitative information on the segmental distribution of function. A low-dose CT provides additional anatomical information to calculate the functional share of the FRL. As described by De Graaf et al. [29], the combination of dynamic HBS with SPECT-CT delivers visible and quantitative information regarding segmental liver function and therefore is an accurate measure of FRL function. The uptake ratio is divided by the body surface area and expressed as $\%/min/m^2$ in order to compensate for differences in individual metabolic requirements. Defining the FRL as ROI enables the estimation of specifically the function of the FRL [19].

The use of $^{99m}$Tc-mebrofenin HBS for the preoperative assessment of liver function in patients undergoing liver surgery was first described by Erdogan et al. [30] and has since been adopted by several hepatobiliary units worldwide [31, 32]. The hepatic uptake of mebrofenin can be calculated in the same way as for ICG. The mebrofenin uptake rate (MUR) strongly correlated with the ICG clearance test. Preoperatively measured FRL function with $^{99m}$Tc-mebrofenin HBS proved to correlate with postoperative FRL function on postoperative day 1 [33]. Furthermore, in patients without parenchymal disease undergoing partial liver resection, preoperative measurement of $^{99m}$Tc-mebrofenin uptake by the FRL was more accurate in predicting postoperative liver insufficiency and liver insufficiency-related mortality than preoperative measurement of FRL volume [34]. In surgical populations with and without compromised liver parenchyma, the MUR cut-off value was calculated at $2.7/min/m^2$, making HBS more valuable in predicting postoperative liver failure compared to CT volumetry [26]. One single cut-off value for patients with compromised or non-compromised livers makes $^{99m}$Tc-mebrofenin HBS an even more suitable liver function test in clinical practice, as the underlying liver disease is often unknown or poorly defined until resection has taken place. Liver biopsies are not routinely taken, as the distribution of compromised parenchyma in the liver is not homogeneous, leading to sampling errors, and because of the risk of biopsy-related complications [35]. This fact increases the value of $^{99m}$Tc-mebrofenin HBS in daily practice. In cholestatic liver disease, however, such as in patients with perihilar cholangiocarcinoma, HBS readings may be affected depending on the completeness of the biliary drainage. Total or segmental MUR will be decreased parallel to and reflecting hyperbilirubinemia as a sign of secondary (obstructive) decreased liver function, which should be taken into consideration [36].

## New Modalities for Assessment of Liver Function

*LiMAx Test ($^{13}$C-Methacetin Breath Test)*

There is a broad spectrum of $^{13}$C-breath tests available. The principle of the $^{13}$C-methacetin breath (LiMAx) test is based on the activity of the cytochrome P450 1A2 (CYP1A2) system, an enzyme system that is exclusively expressed in the liver [37]. The activity of this enzyme system proved to be reduced in patients with severe chronic liver disease regardless of cholestasis. CYP1A2 is distributed throughout the entire functional unit of the liver and is not affected by drugs or genetic variation. $^{13}$C-methacetin, the agent used to measure the activity of CYP1A2, is exclusively metabolized by the CYP1A2 system. $^{13}$C-methacetin is instantly metabolized to paracetamol and ultimately to $^{13}CO_2$, after which $^{13}CO_2$ is excreted through the lungs [38]. This causes alterations in the normal $^{13}CO_2/^{12}CO_2$ ratio in the breath that are analyzed by a modified, non-dispersive, isotope-selective, infrared, spectroscopy-based device. The expired air is collected using a specially designed face mask. In this manner, the $^{13}$C-methacetin breath test provides quantitative information on hepatic function.

The LiMAx test is a non-invasive and easy to perform test, which makes it an attractive option in clinical practice [39]. The cut-off value of normal LiMAx readout is set at 311–575 µg/kg/h. While LiMAx assesses total liver functional capacity, the test can be used to measure FRL function by combining it with CT-volumetric analysis of FRL. The authors assume that the percentage of liver function attributed to the FRL equals the percentage of FRL volume; however, this method does not take into account regional differences in liver function. On the other hand, preoperative FRL LiMAx values correlated with the LiMAx values measured on the first postoperative day. The LiMAx value on postoperative day 1 has also been described as a predictor of PHLF and liver failure-related mortality. The same research group proposed a decision-tree based on the LiMAx results, which is supposed to help surgeons to decide between resection and alternative or additional therapies like PVE, neoadjuvant treatment, and palliative therapy [40]. The value of this algorithm and the proposed cut-off values await further clinical assessment in a prospective setting.

The major limitation of the $^{13}$C-breath tests is the assumption that the contribution of the FRL to total liver function is equal to the proportion of FRL to total liver volume. Inhomogeneous distribution of liver function throughout the liver has been demonstrated using scintigraphic methods as well as with magnetic resonance imaging (MRI) [41, 42]. Another difficulty in the application of the LiMAx test is that the test results are potentially affected by several factors such as hemodialysis, smoking, nutrition, and visceral hemodynamics [40]. Also, members of the CYP1A family are considerably downregulated in HCC, rendering the test less universal in its use for the entire population of patients requiring liver resection [43].

*Assessment of Liver Function Using Magnetic Resonance Imaging*

MRI with gadolinium ethoxybenzyl (Gd-EOB)-DTPA is well established as a liver imaging technique. MRI provides accurate anatomical information and has recently also been introduced as a potential technique for the preoperative assessment of liver function [44–46]. Contrast-enhanced (CE) MRI with Gd-based contrast agents allows a more accurate depiction of benign or malign liver lesions than CT [47].

The concept of using CE-MRI with Gd-EOB-DTPA in the evaluation of liver function was first introduced in 1993 [48]. Subsequently, several studies were published showing a correlation between MRI with Gd-EOB-DTPA and liver function in animal models [49–51]. Recently, data on the assessment of liver function using MRI with Gd-EOB-DTPA in humans were published, all of them confirming the possibility of liver function assessment using MRI [52–54].

Functional imaging with Gd-EOB-DTPA-enhanced MRI has also been used for the assessment of total and regional liver function [55]. Given that MRI now allows the segmental assessment of steatosis and can be used to assess fibrosis, this would make it a potential '1-stop-shop' modality for both liver anatomy and function [56, 57]. However, the use of MRI with Gd-EOB-DTPA for the assessment of liver function is still under investigation. Technical difficulties have to be resolved concerning the molar amount of tracer needed for visualization on MRI, as well as issues regarding the absolute quantification of function.

## Assessment of Increase in FRL Function after PVE

Postoperative regeneration of the remnant liver is usually evaluated by CT volumetry. Failure of the non-embolized liver segments to hypertrophy is considered a significant sign of a deficient functional reserve of the liver, increasing the risk of liver failure associated with liver resection. As postresectional regeneration depends on the same mechanisms, insufficient volume increase of the FRL after PVE is a strong predictor of postoperative liver failure [58, 59].

A decreased ICG clearance rate has been used as a guide when considering preoperative PVE in patients requiring major liver resection in order to augment FRL function. Conceivably, as ICG clearance measures global liver function, an increase in function of the non-embolized lobe is accompanied by decreased function of the embolized atrophied lobe, resulting in no net effect on total liver function. The ICG clearance test is therefore not able to specifically measure the increase in FRL function after PVE.

Scintigraphic techniques are gaining applicability in patients undergoing PVE. Multiple studies evaluated the increase in FRL function after PVE using $^{99m}$Tc-GSA scintigraphy [60–62]. The increase in $^{99m}$Tc-GSA uptake in the FRL was found to be more extensive than the increase in FRL volume. Using $^{99m}$Tc-mebrofenin HBS, it was likewise concluded that the increase in FRL function exceeded the increase in FRL volume [29, 63]. These findings suggest that the time interval between PVE and liver resection may be shorter than determined on the basis of volumetric parameters. Another possible application of HBS in this group of patients is the selection of candidates for PVE or ALPPS. A recent report showed that FRL function assessed with HBS can be used as a predictor of insufficient functional hypertrophy after PVE, especially in non-chemotherapy patients. These patients are potential candidates for upfront ALPPS [64].

The LiMAx test has recently been explored in patients undergoing PVE [65]. In this study, LiMAx was used to visualize the changes in FRL function in the time between PVE and major liver resection, showing an increase in FRL function after PVE. Furthermore, the authors found that FRL function post-resection was lower than the preoperatively calculated function, which they explain by loss of function due to intraoperative injury. The authors recommend that an overestimation margin of the FRL is needed preoperatively in order to compensate for this loss, which renders the test less accurate in this particular setting.

### Assessment of Increase in FRL Function after Stage 1 in ALPPS

In ALPPS, the timing of stage 2, i.e. resection of the deportalized liver lobe, is a much debated issue. The usual imaging modality to assess hypertrophy of the FRL after stage 1 is CT volumetry. As volumetric studies do not consistently correlate with liver function, interstage CT volumetry may be unreliable as a predictor of FRL function in the setting of ALPPS. This notion is corroborated by reports that liver failure after ALPPS stage 2 occurred with an incidence of 30% [66]. Assessment of FRL function therefore seems of great importance for the timing of stage 2. A possible explanation for the discrepancy between volume and function after stage 1 is that hepatocytes after cell division need time to mature before full function can be exerted and that 7–14 days is simply too short a period for function to develop [67].

As discussed above, the ICG clearance test depends on overall liver blood flow and is therefore less applicable during ALPPS because of the division of the portal vein and redistribution of portal and hepatic arterial flow. Furthermore, the ICG clearance test is a global liver function test and does not provide information on specifically segmental function, i.e. the FRL.

Scintigraphic liver function tests such as HBS using $^{99m}$Tc-labeled IDA derivatives have the potential to provide quantitative and visual information on total and regional hepatic function. Sequential measurement of FRL function using HBS therefore seems an advantage in ALPPS. By monitoring inter-stage liver function using HBS, the second stage, i.e. resection of the deportalized lobe, can be safely undertaken [68]. Recently, the use of HBS for the timing of stage 2 in ALPPS was compared with CT volumetry in 60 patients completing ALPPS in 6 European centers. The results showed that volumetry overestimated the liver function [69].

## Discussion

The function of the liver is complex, representing a spectrum of functional processes that can grossly be divided into four categories: uptake, synthesis, biotransformation, and excretion [6]. There is no one functional test that represents the multiple components of liver function, and along the same lines, there is no single test that can accurately predict operative risk in patients considered for major liver resection. We still rely mostly on the combination of clinical parameters and volumetric studies to estimate liver functional reserve and to decide whether we can perform a safe resection. Several techniques are now available for the assessment of liver function of which passive liver tests and dynamic quantitative liver function tests have been employed most frequently. It is time for a change in paradigm, moving from volumetrics to functionometrics in the assessment of surgical risk in patients requiring major liver resection.

Several clinical and quantitative liver function tests have been described in the literature. The Child-Pugh classification, based on clinical symptoms of insufficient liver function (ascites/encephalopathy), and laboratory analysis of parameters of liver function (albumin, bilirubin, and PT) can be used to identify high-risk patients, i.e., class Child B and class Child C. The challenge is, however, to select among class Child A patients those who are good-risk and those who are poor-risk patients [9]. In these patients, reliable quantitative liver function tests are crucial.

Specific liver function tests such as the ICG clearance rate can complement the clinical Child-Pugh classification. The ICG clearance rate has been reported not to unequivocally correlate with morbidity and mortality after partial liver resection. The reported studies, however, vary with respect to the extent of the liver resections performed and the type of patients included (i.e. patients with HCC and cirrhosis vs. patients with normal liver parenchyma). Another drawback of the ICG clearance test is that only global liver function is measured whereas one would be particularly interested in the functional capacity of the part of the liver to be preserved during liver resection. If plasma ICG clearance is multiplied by the proportion of FRL volume, the plasma ICG clearance of specifically the FRL can be calculated. This has been shown to be predictive of PHLF with a cut-off value of 0.05 [70]. This is, however, only applicable in patients with homogenous liver function, making it less feasible in cases of PVE or chronic liver disease.

Nuclear imaging studies have been introduced for the quantitative testing of liver function. Potential advantages of these techniques are the possibility to provide simultaneous morphologic (visual) and physiologic (functional) information of the liver, especially when SPECT-CT cameras are used. Functional capacity may vary within the liver, and with nuclear imaging studies regional differences in hepatic function are detected. SPECT allows measurement of function of specifically the FRL. In addition, when using radiopharmaceutical agents that are excreted into the bile, two dynamic phases can be examined, i.e. hepatic uptake of the agent and secretion into the biliary system. Using $^{99m}$Tc-mebrofenin scintigraphy, definition of a single cut-off value (i.e., 2.7/min/m$^2$) allows the use of a '1-size-fits-all' test to assess non-cholestatic patients irrespective of the quality of liver parenchyma.

Both $^{99m}$Tc-GSA and $^{99m}$Tc-mebrofenin scintigraphy have the potential to preoperatively select patients with a high risk of developing postoperative liver insufficiency who might therefore benefit from PVE. After PVE, hypertrophy of the non-embolized liver segments is commonly monitored by CT volumetry, showing only the morphologic increase in the FRL. However, little is known about the increase in FRL function after PVE with only few available methods to measure FRL function. Although the ICG clearance test is able to measure liver function, this test only quantifies overall liver function and is therefore less suitable for the assessment of post-PVE increase in FRL function. Nuclear imaging studies, however, provide information on augmented function of the FRL. A discrepancy between volumetric hypertrophy and functional increase has been described in several studies, indicating that functional gain of the FRL is more rapid and of greater magnitude than the volumetric increase. Since after PVE the functional advantage of the remnant liver exceeds the volume increase of the residual liver, the recommended waiting time following PVE may be shorter than suggested by volumetric studies [63]. The reverse has been observed in patients undergoing ALPPS in whom in the short time after stage 1 volume exceeds function [69].

There is no one test that can accurately predict the surgical risk in patients considered for major liver resection. Clearly, scoring methods need to be developed in which clinical parameters, CT volumetric criteria, and the results of dynamic quantitative liver function tests guide our decision-making in patients requiring major liver resection. Objective functional criteria are necessary to define patients at increased risk and select those who might benefit from preoperative liver-augmenting techniques.

## Disclosure Statement

The authors have no conflict of interest to disclose.

## References


1 Van den Broek MA, Olde Damink SW, Dejong CH, et al: Liver failure after partial hepatic resection: definition, pathophysiology, risk factors and treatment. Liver Int 2008;28:767–780.
2 Shoup M, Gonen M, D'Angelica M, et al: Volumetric analysis predicts hepatic dysfunction in patients undergoing major liver resection. J Gastrointest Surg 2003; 7:325–330.
3 Vauthey JN, Chaoui A, Do KA, et al: Standardized measurement of the future liver remnant prior to extended liver resection: methodology and clinical associations. Surgery 2000;127:512–519.
4 Martel G, Cieslak KP, Huang R, et al: Comparison of techniques for volumetric analysis of the future liver remnant: implications for major hepatic resections. HPB (Oxford) 2015;17:1051–1057.
5 Field KM, Dow C, Michael M: Part I: Liver function in oncology: biochemistry and beyond. Lancet Oncol 2008;9:1092–1101.
6 Hoekstra LT, de Graaf W, Nibourg GA, et al: Physiological and biochemical basis of clinical liver function tests: a review. Ann Surg 2013;257:27–36.
7 Roberts KJ, Bharathy KG, Lodge JP: Kinetics of liver function tests after a hepatectomy for colorectal liver metastases predict post-operative liver failure as defined by the International Study Group for Liver Surgery. HPB (Oxford) 2013;15:345–351.
8 Nanashima A, Yamaguchi H, Shibasaki S, et al: Measurement of serum hyaluronic acid level during the perioperative period of liver resection for evaluation of functional liver reserve. J Gastroenterol Hepatol 2001; 16:1158–1163.
9 Schneider PD: Preoperative assessment of liver function. Surg Clin North Am 2004;84:355–373.
10 Nagashima I, Takada T, Okinaga K, Nagawa H: A scoring system for the assessment of the risk of mortality after partial hepatectomy in patients with chronic liver dysfunction. J Hepatobiliary Pancreat Surg 2005; 12:44–48.
11 Schroeder RA, Marroquin CE, Bute BP, et al: Predictive indices of morbidity and mortality after liver resection. Ann Surg 2006;243:373–379.
12 Cieslak KP, Runge JH, Heger M, et al: New perspectives in the assessment of future remnant liver. Dig Surg 2014;31:255–268.
13 Paumgartner G: The handling of indocyanine green by the liver. Schweiz Med Wochenschr 1975;105(suppl): 1–30.
14 Okochi O, Kaneko T, Sugimoto H, et al: ICG pulse spectrophotometry for perioperative liver function in hepatectomy. J Surg Res 2002;103:109–113.
15 Akita H, Sasaki Y, Yamada T, et al: Real-time intraoperative assessment of residual liver functional reserve using pulse dye densitometry. World J Surg 2008;32: 2668–2674.
16 Lau H, Man K, Fan ST, et al: Evaluation of preoperative hepatic function in patients with hepatocellular carcinoma undergoing hepatectomy. Br J Surg 1997; 84:1255–1259.
17 Lam CM, Fan ST, Lo CM, Wong J: Major hepatectomy for hepatocellular carcinoma in patients with an unsatisfactory indocyanine green clearance test. Br J Surg 1999;86:1012–1017.
18 Fan ST, Lai EC, Lo CM, et al: Hospital mortality of major hepatectomy for hepatocellular carcinoma associated with cirrhosis. Arch Surg 1995;130:198–203.
19 De Graaf W, Bennink RJ, Veteläinen R, van Gulik TM: Nuclear imaging techniques for the assessment of hepatic function in liver surgery and transplantation. J Nucl Med 2010;51:742–752.
20 Garcea G, Ong SL, Maddern GJ: Predicting liver failure following major hepatectomy. Dig Liver Dis 2009;41: 798–806.
21 Suzuki Y, Kohno Y, Takeda Y, Hiraki Y: Evaluation of liver function parameters by Tc-99m-GSA using multivariate analysis: a study of 47 clinical cases. Acta Med Okayama 1999;53:225–232.
22 Kokudo N, Vera DR, Makuuchi M: Clinical application of TcGSA. Nucl Med Biol 2003;30:845–849.
23 De Graaf W, Häusler S, Heger M, et al: Transporters involved in the hepatic uptake of $^{99m}$Tc-mebrofenin and indocyanine green. J Hepatol 2011;54:738–745.
24 Ghibellini G, Leslie EM, Pollack GM, Brouwer KL: Use of tc-99m mebrofenin as a clinical probe to assess altered hepatobiliary transport: integration of in vitro, pharmacokinetic modeling, and simulation studies. Pharm Res 2008;25:1851–1860.
25 Trauner M, Meier PJ, Boyer JL: Molecular pathogenesis of cholestasis. N Engl J Med 1998;339:1217–1227.
26 De Graaf W, van Lienden KP, Dinant S, et al: Assessment of future remnant liver function using hepatobiliary scintigraphy in patients undergoing major liver resection. J Gastrointest Surg 2010;14:369–378.
27 Cieslak KP, Bennink RJ, de Graaf W, et al: Measurement of liver function using hepatobiliary scintigraphy improves risk assessment in patients undergoing major liver resection. HPB (Oxford) 2016;18:773–780.
28 Ekman M, Fjälling M, Friman S, et al: Liver uptake function measured by IODIDA clearance rate in liver transplant patients and healthy volunteers. Nucl Med Commun 1996;17:235–242.
29 De Graaf W, van Lienden KP, van Gulik TM, Bennink RJ: $^{99m}$Tc-mebrofenin hepatobiliary scintigraphy with SPECT for the assessment of hepatic function and liver functional volume before partial hepatectomy. J Nucl Med 2010;51:229–236.
30 Erdogan D, Heijnen BH, Bennink RJ, et al: Preoperative assessment of liver function: a comparison of 99mTc-mebrofenin scintigraphy with indocyanine green clearance test. Liver Int 2004;24:117–123.
31 Serenari M, Collaud C, Alvarez FA, et al: Interstage assessment of remnant liver function in ALPPS using hepatobiliary scintigraphy: prediction of posthepatectomy liver failure and introduction of the HIBA index. Ann Surg 2017;DOI: 10.1097/SLA.0000000000002150.
32 Chapelle T, Op De Beeck B, Huyghe I, et al: Future remnant liver function estimated by combining liver volumetry on magnetic resonance imaging with total liver function on $^{99m}$Tc-mebrofenin hepatobiliary scintigraphy: can this tool predict post-hepatectomy liver failure? HPB (Oxford) 2016;18:494–503.
33 Bennink RJ, Dinant S, Erdogan D, et al: Preoperative assessment of postoperative remnant liver function using hepatobiliary scintigraphy. J Nucl Med 2004;45: 965–971.
34 Dinant S, de Graaf W, Verwer BJ, et al: Risk assessment of posthepatectomy liver failure using hepatobiliary scintigraphy and CT volumetry. J Nucl Med 2007; 48:685–692.
35 Ratziu V, Charlotte F, Heurtier A, et al: Sampling variability of liver biopsy in nonalcoholic fatty liver disease. Gastroenterology 2005;128:1898–1906.

36 Olthof PB, Coelen RJS, Bennink RJ, et al: 99mTc-mebrofenin hepatobiliary scintigraphy predicts liver failure following major liver resection for perihilar cholangiocarcinoma. HPB (Oxford) 2017;19:850–858.
37 Guengerich FP, Krauser JA, Johnson WW: Rate-limiting steps in oxidations catalyzed by rabbit cytochrome P450 1A2. Biochemistry 2004;43:10775–10788.
38 Schoeller DA, Schneider JF, Solomons NW, et al: Clinical diagnosis with the stable isotope 13C in $CO_2$ breath tests: methodology and fundamental considerations. J Lab Clin Med 1977;90:412–421.
39 Stockmann M, Lock JF, Riecke B, et al: Prediction of postoperative outcome after hepatectomy with a new bedside test for maximal liver function capacity. Ann Surg 2009;250:119–125.
40 Stockmann M, Lock JF, Malinowski M, et al: The LiMAx test: a new liver function test for predicting postoperative outcome in liver surgery. HPB (Oxford) 2010;12:139–146.
41 Sumiyoshi T, Shima Y, Tokorodani R, et al: CT/99mTc-GSA SPECT fusion images demonstrate functional differences between the liver lobes. World J Gastroenterol 2013;19:3217–3225.
42 Nilsson H, Karlgren S, Blomqvist L, Jonas E: The inhomogeneous distribution of liver function: possible impact on the prediction of post-operative remnant liver function. HPB (Oxford) 2015;17:272–277.
43 McKinnon RA, Hall PD, Quattrochi LC, et al: Localization of CYP1A1 and CYP1A2 messenger RNA in normal human liver and in hepatocellular carcinoma by in situ hybridization. Hepatology 1991;14:848–856.
44 Nilsson H, Nordell A, Vargas R, et al: Assessment of hepatic extraction fraction and input relative blood flow using dynamic hepatocyte-specific contrast-enhanced MRI. J Magn Reson Imaging 2009;29:1323–1331.
45 Sourbron S, Sommer WH, Reiser MF, Zech CJ: Combined quantification of liver perfusion and function with dynamic gadoxetic acid-enhanced MR imaging. Radiology 2012;263:874–883.
46 Saito K, Ledsam J, Sourbron S, et al: Measuring hepatic functional reserve using low temporal resolution Gd-EOB-DTPA dynamic contrast-enhanced MRI: a preliminary study comparing galactosyl human serum albumin scintigraphy with indocyanine green retention. Eur Radiol 2014;24:112–119.
47 Niekel MC, Bipat S, Stoker J: Diagnostic imaging of colorectal liver metastases with CT, MR imaging, FDG PET, and/or FDG PET/CT: a meta-analysis of prospective studies including patients who have not previously undergone treatment. Radiology 2010;257:674–684.
48 Schuhmann-Giampieri G: Liver contrast media for magnetic resonance imaging. Interrelations between pharmacokinetics and imaging. Invest Radiol 1993;28:753–761.
49 Ryeom HK, Kim SH, Kim JY, et al: Quantitative evaluation of liver function with MRI using Gd-EOB-DTPA. Korean J Radiol 2004;5:231–239.
50 Tsuda N, Okada M, Murakami T: New proposal for the staging of nonalcoholic steatohepatitis: evaluation of liver fibrosis on Gd-EOB-DTPA-enhanced MRI. Eur J Radiol 2010;73:137–142.
51 Tsuda N, Okada M, Murakami T: Potential of gadolinium-ethoxybenzyl-diethylenetriamine pentaacetic acid (Gd-EOB-DTPA) for differential diagnosis of nonalcoholic steatohepatitis and fatty liver in rats using magnetic resonance imaging. Invest Radiol 2007;42:242–247.
52 Nilsson H, Blomqvist L, Douglas L, et al: Gd-EOB-DTPA-enhanced MRI for the assessment of liver function and volume in liver cirrhosis. Br J Radiol 2013;86:20120653.
53 Motosugi U, Ichikawa T, Sou H, et al: Liver parenchymal enhancement of hepatocyte-phase images in Gd-EOB-DTPA-enhanced MR imaging: which biological markers of the liver function affect the enhancement? J Magn Reson Imaging 2009;30:1042–1046.
54 Tajima T, Takao H, Akai H, et al: Relationship between liver function and liver signal intensity in hepatobiliary phase of gadolinium ethoxybenzyl diethylenetriamine pentaacetic acid-enhanced magnetic resonance imaging. J Comput Assist Tomogr 2010;34:362–366.
55 Nilsson H, Blomqvist L, Douglas L, et al: Assessment of liver function in primary biliary cirrhosis using Gd-EOB-DTPA-enhanced liver MRI. HPB (Oxford) 2010;12:567–576.
56 Van Werven JR, Marsman HA, Nederveen AJ, et al: Assessment of hepatic steatosis in patients undergoing liver resection: comparison of US, CT, T1-weighted dual-echo MR imaging, and point-resolved 1H MR spectroscopy. Radiology 2010;256:159–168.
57 Venkatesh SK, Yin M, Ehman RL: Magnetic resonance elastography of liver: technique, analysis, and clinical applications. J Magn Reson Imaging 2013;37:544–555.
58 Ribero D, Abdalla EK, Madoff DC, et al: Portal vein embolization before major hepatectomy and its effects on regeneration, resectability and outcome. Br J Surg 2007;94:1386–1394.
59 Van Gulik TM, van den Esschert JW, de Graaf W, et al: Controversies in the use of portal vein embolization. Dig Surg 2008;25:436–444.
60 Hirai I, Kimura W, Fuse A, et al: Evaluation of preoperative portal embolization for safe hepatectomy, with special reference to assessment of nonembolized lobe function with 99mTc-GSA SPECT scintigraphy. Surgery 2003;133:495–506.
61 Nishiyama Y, Yamamoto Y, Hino I, et al: $^{99m}$Tc galactosyl human serum albumin liver dynamic SPET for pre-operative assessment of hepatectomy in relation to percutaneous transhepatic portal embolization. Nucl Med Commun 2003;24:809–817.
62 Nanashima A, Yamaguchi H, Shibasaki S, et al: Relationship between CT volumetry and functional liver volume using technetium-99m galactosyl serum albumin scintigraphy in patients undergoing preoperative portal vein embolization before major hepatectomy: a preliminary study. Dig Dis Sci 2006;51:1190–1195.
63 De Graaf W, van Lienden KP, van den Esschert JW, et al: Increase in future remnant liver function after preoperative portal vein embolization. Br J Surg 2011;98:825–834.
64 Cieslak KP, Huisman F, Bais T, et al: Future remnant liver function as predictive factor for the hypertrophy response after portal vein embolization. Surgery 2017;162:37–47.
65 Malinowski M, Lock JF, Seehofer D, et al: Preliminary study on liver function changes after trisectionectomy with versus without prior portal vein embolization. Surg Today 2016;46:1053–1061.
66 Schadde E, Raptis DA, Schnitzbauer AA, et al: Prediction of mortality after ALPPS stage-1: an analysis of 320 patients from the International ALPPS Registry. Ann Surg 2015;262:780–785; discussion 785–786.
67 Matsuo K, Murakami T, Kawaguchi D, et al: Histologic features after surgery associating liver partition and portal vein ligation for staged hepatectomy versus those after hepatectomy with portal vein embolization. Surgery 2016;159:1289–1298.
68 Cieslak KP, Olthof PB, van Lienden KP, et al: Assessment of liver function using $^{99m}$Tc-mebrofenin hepatobiliary scintigraphy in ALPPS (associating liver partition and portal vein ligation for staged hepatectomy). Case Rep Gastroenterol 2015;9:353–360.
69 Olthof PB, Tomassini F, Huespe PE, et al: Hepatobiliary scintigraphy to evaluate liver function in associating liver partition and portal vein ligation for staged hepatectomy: liver volume overestimates liver function. Surgery 2017;162:775–783.
70 Yokoyama Y, Nishio H, Ebata T, et al: Value of indocyanine green clearance of the future liver remnant in predicting outcome after resection for biliary cancer. Br J Surg 2010;97:1260–1268.

Visceral Medicine

**Review Article**

Visc Med 2017;33:449–454
DOI: 10.1159/000479046

Published online: November 22, 2017

# ICG Clearance Test and 99mTc-GSA SPECT/CT Fusion Images

Yuji Iimuro

Department of Surgery, Hepato-Biliary-Pancreatic Disease Center, Yamanashi Prefectural Central Hospital, Yamanashi, Japan

**Keywords**
Liver function · Indocyanine green · GSA SPECT

**Summary**
Preoperative estimation of future remnant liver function is critical for major hepatic surgery to avoid postoperative morbidity and mortality. Among several liver function tests, the indocyanine green (ICG) clearance test is still the most popular dynamic method. The usefulness of ICG clearance test parameters, such as ICGR15, $K_{ICG}$, or $PDR_{ICG}$, has been reported by many investigators. The transcutaneous non-invasive pulse dye densitometry system has made the ICG clearance test more convenient and attractive, even in Western countries. The concept of future remnant $K_{ICG}$ (rem $K_{ICG}$), which combines the functional aspect and the volumetric factor of the future remnant liver, seems ideal for determining the maximum extent of major hepatic resection that will not cause postoperative liver failure. For damaged livers with functional heterogeneity among the hepatic segments, fusion images combining technetium-99m-diethylenetriaminepentaacetic acid-galactosyl human serum albumin single photon emission computed tomography (99mTc-GSA SPECT) and X-ray CT are helpful to precisely estimate the functional reserve of the future remnant liver. Another technique for image-based liver function estimation, gadolinium ethoxybenzyl diethylenetriamine pentaacetic acid(Gd-EOB)-enhanced magnetic resonance imaging, may be an ideal candidate for the preoperative determination of future remnant liver function. Using these methods effectively, morbidity and mortality after major hepatic resection could be reduced.



## Introduction

The preoperative estimation of future remnant liver function is essential for extensive liver resection to avoid postoperative morbidity and mortality. Estimation of remaining liver volume is the first step in creating a surgical plan. The hepatic circulation-based 3-dimensional (3D) hepatectomy simulation system, which was first reported in 2005, has largely contributed to the accurate assessment of the remaining liver volume [1]. This kind of computer-assisted volumetry allows the precise calculation of either the ratio of remnant liver volume to total liver volume (RLV/TLV) or the ratio of remnant liver volume to body weight (RLV/BW). Using these ratios, several investigators have reported safe thresholds to prevent postoperative liver failure in non-cirrhotic patients [2–4]. However, a more cautious assessment of the functional aspects of remnant liver is required in patients with underlying liver disease such as cirrhosis, or in patients with impaired liver function due to chemotherapy for liver metastasis from colorectal cancer [5, 6]. In addition, portal vein embolization (PVE) or associating liver partition and portal vein ligation for staged hepatectomy (ALPPS) have been employed for extensive liver resection to avoid postoperative complications by inducing hypertrophy of the future remnant liver. In these methods, especially in ALPPS, a discrepancy between the volumetric increase and the functional improvement in the future remnant liver has been reported [7–9].

For the assessment of preoperative liver function, static and dynamic tests are available. The Child-Turcotte-Pugh (CTP) [10, 11] and model for end-stage liver disease (MELD) [12, 13] scoring systems are well-known methods for the static assessment of liver function and are useful for predicting postoperative morbidity and mortality [14–17]. However, static laboratory tests are sometimes insensitive at predicting postoperative liver functional reserve. Thus, dynamic liver function tests have been used in deciding about the operability of patients with underlying liver disease. The preoperative estimation of future remnant liver function is especially critical in patients with functional heterogeneity among the

KARGER

Fax +49 761 4 52 07 14
Information@Karger.com
www.karger.com



Accessible online at:
www.karger.com/vis

Yuji Iimuro, MD, PhD
Department of Surgery, Hepato-Biliary-Pancreatic Disease Center
Yamanashi Prefectural Central Hospital
1-1-1 Fujimi, Kofu, Yamanashi, 400-8506, Japan
siimuro@hyo-med.ac.jp

**Table 1.** Indocyanine green (ICG) clearance test parameters in the assessment of hepatic function

| | Description | Calculation | Unit |
|---|---|---|---|
| ICGR15 | ICG retention ratio after 15 min | $(C_{ICG\,(15)} / C_{ICG\,(0)}) \times 100$ | % |
| $K_{ICG}$ | rate constant (k) of ICG indicator-dilution curve | $C_{ICG\,(t)} = C_{ICG\,(0)} \times e^{-kt}$ | $min^{-1}$ |
| $PDR_{ICG}$ | plasma disappearance rate of ICG | $K_{ICG} \times 100$ | % $min^{-1}$ |

$C_{ICG\,(t)}$ = ICG concentration at time point t [34]; k = fractional ICG concentration change per minute; e = Euler's number.

hepatic segments. Thus, for the evaluation of the effectiveness of PVE or ALPPS, dynamic liver function tests which can estimate spatial functional distribution in the liver are required. Among several dynamic tests, the indocyanine green (ICG) clearance test and fusion images of technetium-99m-diethylenetriaminepentaacetic acid-galactosyl human serum albumin single photon emission computed tomography (99mTc-GSA SPECT)/X-ray computed tomography (CT) are discussed in this review.

## ICG Clearance Test

The ICG clearance test has been the most popular dynamic liver function test, especially in Eastern countries. ICG is a non-toxic, inert, anionic water-soluble tricarbocyanide dye, first introduced by Fox and Brooker for the assessment of cardiac output [18]. Soon after, the usefulness of this dye for assessing liver function and hepatic blood flow was reported by several investigators [19, 20]. ICG administered intravenously is almost exclusively extracted by the liver, and its elimination is dependent on hepatocyte function, liver blood flow, and bile secretion. Thus, the ICG clearance test is considered to accurately correlate with hepatic function and has been widely used in clinical settings in Eastern countries for a long time.

The standard method for quantifying hepatic ICG clearance is ex-vivo photometric analysis of consecutive blood samples obtained within a 15-min frame after intravenous bolus injection [19, 20]. The absolute clearance of ICG or the fractional change per minute can be calculated from a concentration-time curve obtained. This method is accurate and reproducible, but has not been widely adopted in Western countries because of its invasiveness and complexity. Transcutaneous non-invasive pulse dye densitometry (PDD), which was first invented by Aoyagi who is also known for the invention of pulse oximetry [21, 22], is now commercially available in both Western and Eastern countries. Two PDD systems for the ICG clearance test are available: the LiMON device (Pulsion Medical System, Munich, Germany) and the DDG-3000 analyzer (Nihon-Kohden, Tokyo, Japan). Both devices calculate ICG retention 15 (ICGR15; the ICG retention ratio after 15 min) and the rate constant (k) of the indicator-dilution curve using backward dynamic extrapolation ($K_{ICG}$). The k value is then multiplied by 100 to obtain the plasma disappearance rate of ICG ($PDR_{ICG}$). Acceptable accuracy of the PDD system has been reported after comparing data derived from invasive and non-invasive methods [23–27]. These non-invasive PDD systems have made the ICG clearance test more attractive even in Western countries, and many investigators have recently reported its usefulness as a non-invasive dynamic liver function test [28–31].

### *ICGR 15*

ICGR15 is the ratio between the ICG concentration 15 min after injection and the initial concentration; ICGR15 (%) = $C_{ICG\,(15)} / C_{ICG\,(0)} \times 100$ (table 1). ICGR15 has been widely used as an alternative to $K_{ICG}$ or $PDR_{ICG}$ because of its relative convenience. $K_{ICG}$ or $PDR_{ICG}$ require serial blood sampling and ex-vivo photometric analysis using a standard invasive method, while ICGR15 can be calculated from one-point sampling at 15 min. Clinical data concerning preoperative ICGR15 and postoperative liver failure have been accumulated from the early 1980s [32–38], and a decision tree for the hepatectomy procedure, which includes ICGR15 as a parameter in addition to the presence or absence of ascites and the serum total bilirubin level, has been proposed [39]. Very low mortality has been reported using the decision tree for the hepatectomy procedure [40], and the use of ICGR15 was recommended for the preoperative assessment of liver function in the evidence-based clinical guidelines for the diagnosis and treatment of hepatocellular carcinoma in Japan [41].

### *$PDR_{ICG}$ or $K_{ICG}$*

The plasma disappearance rate of ICG ($PDR_{ICG}$; % per minute) is the percentage change over the time of the reduction in ICG blood concentration starting from a concentration of 100%. The rate constant (k) of the ICG indicator-dilution curve ($K_{ICG}$) can be calculated using backward dynamic extrapolation of the elimination phase $C_{ICG}$ (t) = $C_0 \times e^{-kt}$. The k value is then multiplied by 100 to obtain the $PDR_{ICG}$ as a percentage per minute (table 1). $K_{ICG}$ or $PDR_{ICG}$ have been thought to reflect the pharmacokinetics of ICG more accurately than ICGR15 because the former require multiple sampling time points. However, $K_{ICG}$ or $PDR_{ICG}$ had not been widely used worldwide, except in Japan, because of the complexity of the method. After the non-invasive PDD systems became commercially available, many investigators reported the usefulness of these parameters to assess perioperative liver function [30] and even more so to predict the prognosis of critically ill patients [42–45].

### *Rem $K_{ICG}$*

The preoperative estimation of liver function employing ICGR15, $PDR_{ICG}$, or $K_{ICG}$ is important for obvious reasons. However, how well the future remnant liver will actually function after hepatic resection is a much more interesting issue for liver surgeons. Namely, it is critical to assess the maximum extent of major hepatic resection that will not cause postoperative liver failure. The concept of future remnant $K_{ICG}$ (rem $K_{ICG}$), which is calculated from the preoperative $K_{ICG}$ and the proportion of the future remnant liver volume to the whole functional liver parenchymal volume (rem $K_{ICG}$ = preoperative $K_{ICG}$ × proportion of the future liver remnant), was first proposed by Takasaki et al. [32]. This concept of combining the functional aspect and the volumetric factor of the liver seems ideal for predicting postoperative liver function after extended liver resection, despite its complexity. Takasaki et al. [32] proposed that rem $K_{ICG} > 0.062$ is a safety threshold for postoperative mortality [32]. Other investigators also reported that postoperative morbidity was low in patients with rem $K_{ICG} > 0.06$ after a major hepatectomy [46], or that rem $K_{ICG} \geq 0.05$ was a threshold for survival in patients with bile duct cancer who underwent preoperative PVE [47]. More recently, on the basis of statistical analysis, a rem $K_{ICG}$ of 0.05 has been again reported as a useful cut-off value for predicting mortality and morbidity in patients with biliary cancer [48, 49]. On the other hand, morbidity was 100% in a rem $K_{ICG}$ range of < 0.03 [46], indicating that in patients with rem $K_{ICG}$ below 0.03 liver resection is contraindicated.

After the non-invasive PDD systems became available and a real-time and rapid ICG clearance test was possible, intraoperative estimation of remnant liver function by trial clamping of selective arterial and portovenous inflow was reported [29, 50, 51]. In addition, early prediction of postoperative liver dysfunction using real-time $PDR_{ICG}$ has also been proposed after major liver resection [30, 52] or liver transplantation [53–55]. Recent advances in the 3D CT volumetric system in combination with non-invasive PDD systems have made accurate calculation of rem $K_{ICG}$ easier. Thus, the non-invasive ICG clearance test has become a more attractive and convenient modality.

*Limitations of the ICG Clearance Test*

The ICG clearance test is a reliable dynamic liver function test but has some limitations. First, ICG elimination should be interpreted with caution in patients with cholestasis. Bilirubin and ICG competitively bind to the same organic anion transporting polypeptides such as 1B3 (OATP 1B3) [56], possibly leading to a reduced uptake of ICG in patients with obstructive jaundice. This condition could also be observed in the early postoperative period after liver transplantation in patients with pretransplant hyperbilirubinemia. The usefulness of the LiMAx test, another dynamic liver function test, is also reported in Western countries [8, 57, 58]. The LiMAx test evaluates whole liver function, detecting the $^{13}CO_2/^{12}CO_2$ ratio in expired air, which depends on the rate of metabolization of $^{13}$C-methacetin by P450 1A2 (CYP1A2) in hepatocytes [57]. While LiMAx, as a whole liver function test, is similar to the ICG clearance test, it can be used independent of cholestasis. However, the LiMAx test requires specialized equipment to detect $^{13}$C, and is expensive. Therefore, it should be cautiously observed whether the LiMAx test really possesses significant advantage over the ICG clearance test. Portal flow is also an important factor affecting ICG clearance. In patients with giant splenorenal shunt, specifically decreased ICG clearance values are often observed compared to other liver functional parameters. In patients with constitutional ICG excretory defect [59], the ICG clearance test is also not efficient.

## GSA-SPECT Fusion Image

The ICG clearance test is still a gold standard dynamic method to assess liver function as mentioned above. Rem $K_{ICG}$, which combines the volumetric factor of the remnant liver and ICG pharmacokinetics, is an ideal concept in a situation where the functional distribution is supposed to be homogeneous throughout the liver. However, functional heterogeneity among the hepatic segments often exists in a damaged liver, cirrhotic liver, liver after PVE, or liver with portal tumor thrombus. Such situations require other dynamic liver function tests that can estimate spatial functional distribution in the liver.

The asialoglycoprotein receptor (ASGPR) is located on the sinusoidal surface of hepatocytes and is involved in the clearance of glycoproteins containing terminal galactose residues from the circulation [60]. Vera et al. [61–63] first reported ASGPR-mediated binding of 99mTc-galactosyl-neoglycoalbumin (99mTc-NGA) in vitro and in vivo. In addition, a decrease in hepatic ASGPR expression has been reported in patients with liver damage [64]. Thus, analysis of ASGPR expression has been widely performed using 99mTc-GSA, an analog of asialoglycoproteins, to estimate liver function in damaged livers [65–69]. For example, a receptor index parameter (LHL15), obtained from the liver and heart time-activity data as the ratio of radioactivity of the liver over that of the liver plus heart at 15 min after intravenous injection of Tc-GSA correlated well with classical indicators for hepatic functional capacity such as the serum albumin level, serum bilirubin level, prothrombin time, ICGR15, or CTP criteria score [65, 70].

Moreover, 99mTc-GSA SPECT, which enables the evaluation of regional GSA accumulation in the liver, was developed to precisely investigate the regional distribution of hepatic function [71–73]. There are several 99mTc-GSA SPECT parameters such as the liver uptake ratio (LUR) [74, 75], liver uptake density [74, 76], liver uptake value corrected for body surface area (LUV) [77], or uptake index [78, 79]; all these parameters basically depend on the regional strength of radioactivity in the liver. The parameter LUR correlates well with the extent of ASGPR expression immunohistochemically evaluated, and a parallel decrease in LUR and ASGPR protein expression was observed in the fibrotic liver [80]. It is noteworthy that functional heterogeneity among hepatic segments has been reported in damaged liver by employing 99mTc-GSA SPECT [72, 81, 82], suggesting its usefulness for the precise prediction of postoperative hepatic functional reserve in the damaged liver.

Recent advances in X-ray CT systems, including 3D CT simulation [1], have made precise preoperative surgical planning for liver resection easier. Therefore, fusion images combining 99mTc-GSA SPECT and X-ray CT could be critically helpful for preoperative surgical decision making [80, 83–86]. Accordingly, future remnant liver function has been estimated on the fusion images, calculating the strength of radioactivity in the future remnant hepatic area (fig. 1), and expressed as remnant LUR [80], remnant LUV [87], R0-remnant [83], or functional hepatic resection rate (FURR) [86]. Even though these methods have not been widely accepted in clinical practice worldwide because of their complexity, they are especially useful in patients with regional heterogeneity of liver function, that is, patients who undergo preoperative PVE for insufficient remnant liver volume [7, 74, 88] or who receive bile duct drainage for obstructive jaundice due to bile duct cancer [89]. In these contexts, 99mTc-GSA SPECT/X-ray CT fusion images are supposed to be useful for the evaluation of the effectiveness of ALPPS in terms of hepatocyte proliferation and function in the future remnant liver.

In European countries, hepatobiliary scintigraphy (HBS) using 99mTc-mebrofenin is often employed to estimate spatial functional distribution in the liver [90–94]. Upon intravenous administration, 99mTc-mebrofenin is extracted exclusively by the hepatocytes, and excreted in the bile via the ATP-dependent export pump. The transporter of 99mTc-mebrofenin and ICG partially overlaps [56]. Thus, 99mTc-mebrofenin HBS relies on pharmacokinetics similar to those of the ICG clearance test, and is mechanistically completely different from 99mTc-GSA SPECT. From the view point of the increase in the number of hepatocytes, 99mTc-GSA SPECT may possibly be more suitable for evaluating functional improvement in the future remnant liver after PVE or ALPPS.

Fusion images combining 99mTc-GSA SPECT and X-ray CT are a theoretically rational method, and its clinical usefulness has been reported as mentioned above. However, this method has not been in widespread use in Western countries because of its complexity and equipment requirements. Another technique for image-based liver function estimation, gadolinium ethoxybenzyl diethylenetriamine pentaacetic acid(Gd-EOB-DTPA)-enhanced magnetic resonance imaging (MRI), could be an ideal candidate for the preoperative determination of liver function [95]. Gd-EOB-enhanced MRI can display regional liver function with good spatial resolution, which is critically useful for preoperative surgical decisions. For the evaluation of its usefulness as a liver functional test, the best conditional setting and the interpretation of the acquired data are currently under investigation [76].

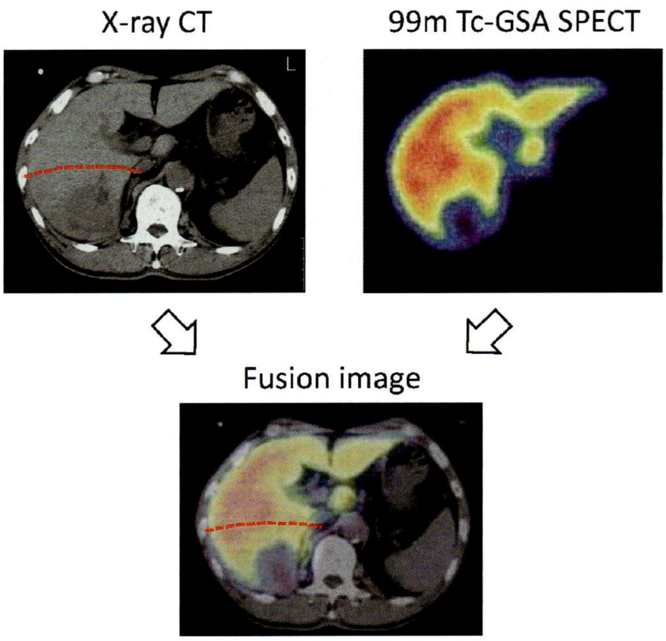


**Fig. 1.** Fusion images combining X-ray computed tomography (CT) and technetium-99m-diethylenetriaminepentaacetic acid-galactosyl human serum albumin single photon emission computed tomography (99mTc-GSA SPECT). The strength of radioactivity in the future remnant liver can be accurately estimated on the fusion images (lower) combining X-ray CT (upper left) and 99mTc-GSA SPECT (upper right).

## Conclusion

The ICG clearance test remains the most popular dynamic liver function test and has become a more convenient method after non-invasive PDD systems were made available. According to safety criteria employing ICGR15, $PDR_{ICG}$, or $K_{ICG}$, morbidity and mortality after major hepatic resection can be reduced. For patients with functional heterogeneity among the liver segments, fusion images combining 99mTc-GSA SPECT and X-ray CT are useful to precisely predict future remnant liver function. Gd-EOB-enhanced MRI could also become an ideal candidate for imaging-based liver function tests.

## Disclosure Statement

The author declares that he has nothing to disclose representing a potential conflict of interest with respect to this manuscript.

## References

1 Saito S, Yamanaka J, Miura K, Nakao N, Nagao T, Sugimoto T, Hirano T, Kuroda N, Iimuro Y, Fujimoto J: A novel 3D hepatectomy simulation based on liver circulation: application to liver resection and transplantation. Hepatology 2005;41:1297–1304.

2 Chun YS, Ribero D, Abdalla EK, Madoff DC, Mortenson MM, Wei SH, Vauthey JN: Comparison of two methods of future liver remnant volume measurement. J Gastrointest Surg 2008;12:123–128.

3 Truant S, Oberlin O, Sergent G, Lebuffe G, Gambiez L, Ernst O, Pruvot FR: Remnant liver volume to body weight ratio ≥0.5%: a new cut-off to estimate postoperative risks after extended resection in noncirrhotic liver. J Am Coll Surg 2007;204:22–33.

4 Yigitler C, Farges O, Kianmanesh R, Regimbeau JM, Abdalla EK, Belghiti J: The small remnant liver after major liver resection: how common and how relevant? Liver Transpl 2003;9:S18–25.

5 Narita M, Oussoultzoglou E, Fuchshuber P, Pessaux P, Chenard MP, Rosso E, Nobili C, Jaeck D, Bachellier P: What is a safe future liver remnant size in patients undergoing major hepatectomy for colorectal liver metastases and treated by intensive preoperative chemotherapy? Ann Surg Oncol 2012;19:2526–2538.

6 Shindoh J, Tzeng CW, Aloia TA, Curley SA, Zimmitti G, Wei SH, Huang SY, Mahvash A, Gupta S, Wallace MJ, Vauthey JN: Optimal future liver remnant in patients treated with extensive preoperative chemotherapy for colorectal liver metastases. Ann Surg Oncol 2013;20:2493–2500.
7 Hirai I, Kimura W, Fuse A, Suto K, Urayama M: Evaluation of preoperative portal embolization for safe hepatectomy, with special reference to assessment of nonembolized lobe function with 99mTc-GSA SPECT scintigraphy. Surgery 2003;133:495–506.
8 Malinowski M, Lock JF, Seehofer D, Gebauer B, Schulz A, Demirel L, Bednarsch J, Stary V, Neuhaus P, Stockmann M: Preliminary study on liver function changes after trisectionectomy with versus without prior portal vein embolization. Surg Today 2016;46:1053–1061.
9 Olthof PB, Schadde E, van Lienden KP, Heger M, de Bruin K, Verheij J, Bennink RJ, van Gulik TM: Hepatic parenchymal transection increases liver volume but not function after portal vein embolization in rabbits. Surgery 2017;162:732–741.
10 Child CG, Turcotte JG: Surgery and portal hypertension. Major Probl Clin Surg 1964;1:1–85.
11 Pugh RN, Murray-Lyon IM, Dawson JL, Pietroni MC, Williams R: Transection of the oesophagus for bleeding oesophageal varices. Br J Surg 1973;60:646–649.
12 Malinchoc M, Kamath PS, Gordon FD, Peine CJ, Rank J, ter Borg PC: A model to predict poor survival in patients undergoing transjugular intrahepatic portosystemic shunts. Hepatology 2000;31:864–871.
13 Cholongitas E, Marelli L, Shusang V, Senzolo M, Rolles K, Patch D, Burroughs AK: A systematic review of the performance of the model for end-stage liver disease (MELD) in the setting of liver transplantation. Liver Transpl 2006;12:1049–1061.
14 Vauthey JN, Klimstra D, Franceschi D, Tao Y, Fortner J, Blumgart L, Brennan M: Factors affecting long-term outcome after hepatic resection for hepatocellular carcinoma. Am J Surg 1995;169:28–34; discussion 34–35.
15 Teh SH, Christein J, Donohue J, Que F, Kendrick M, Farnell M, Cha S, Kamath P, Kim R, Nagorney DM: Hepatic resection of hepatocellular carcinoma in patients with cirrhosis: Model of End-Stage Liver Disease (MELD) score predicts perioperative mortality. J Gastrointest Surg 2005;9:1207–1215; discussion 1215.
16 Cucchetti A, Ercolani G, Vivarelli M, Cescon M, Ravaioli M, La Barba G, Zanello M, Grazi GL, Pinna AD: Impact of model for end-stage liver disease (MELD) score on prognosis after hepatectomy for hepatocellular carcinoma on cirrhosis. Liver Transpl 2006;12:966–971.
17 Delis SG, Bakoyiannis A, Biliatis I, Athanassiou K, Tassopoulos N, Dervenis C: Model for end-stage liver disease (MELD) score, as a prognostic factor for post-operative morbidity and mortality in cirrhotic patients, undergoing hepatectomy for hepatocellular carcinoma. HPB (Oxford) 2009;11:351–357.
18 Fox IJ, Brooker LG, Heseltine DW, Essex HE, Wood EH: A tricarbocyanine dye for continuous recording of dilution curves in whole blood independent of variations in blood oxygen saturation. Proc Staff Meet Mayo Clin 1957;32:478–484.
19 Cherrick GR, Stein SW, Leevy CM, Davidson CS: Indocyanine green: observations on its physical properties, plasma decay, and hepatic extraction. J Clin Invest 1960;39:592–600.
20 Wiegand BD, Ketterer SG, Rapaport E: The use of indocyanine green for the evaluation of hepatic function and blood flow in man. Am J Dig Dis 1960;5:427–436.
21 Aoyagi T, Kishi M, Yamaguchi K, Watanable S: Improvement of the earpiece oximeter; in: Abstracts of the 13th Annual Meeting of the Japanese Society for Medical Electronics and Biological Engineering. Osaka, 1974, pp 90–91.
22 Aoyagi T, Kishi M, Yamaguchi K, Nakajima S, Hirai H, Takase H: New pulse-type ear oximeter. Kokyu To Juncan 1975;23:709–713.
23 Ishigami Y, Masuzawa M, Miyoshi E, et al: Clinical applications of ICG Finger Monitor in patients with liver disease. J Hepatol 1993;19:232–240.
24 Tsubono T, Todo S, Jabbour N, Mizoe A, Warty V, Demetris AJ, Starzl TE: Indocyanine green elimination test in orthotopic liver recipients. Hepatology 1996;24:1165–1171.
25 Sakka SG, Reinhart K, Meier-Hellmann A: Comparison of invasive and noninvasive measurements of indocyanine green plasma disappearance rate in critically ill patients with mechanical ventilation and stable hemodynamics. Intensive Care Med 2000;26:1553–1556.
26 Faybik P, Krenn CG, Baker A, Lahner D, Berlakovich G, Steltzer H, Hetz H: Comparison of invasive and noninvasive measurement of plasma disappearance rate of indocyanine green in patients undergoing liver transplantation: a prospective investigator-blinded study. Liver Transpl 2004;10:1060–1064.
27 Sakka SG, van Hout N: Relation between indocyanine green (ICG) plasma disappearance rate and ICG blood clearance in critically ill patients. Intensive Care Med 2006;32:766–769.
28 Krieger PM, Tamandl D, Herberger B, Faybik P, Fleischmann E, Maresch J, Gruenberger T: Evaluation of chemotherapy-associated liver injury in patients with colorectal cancer liver metastases using indocyanine green clearance testing. Ann Surg Oncol 2011;18:1644–1650.
29 Thomas MN, Weninger E, Angele M, Bosch F, Pratschke S, Andrassy J, Rentsch M, Stangl M, Hartwig W, Werner J, Guba M: Intraoperative simulation of remnant liver function during anatomic liver resection with indocyanine green clearance (LiMON) measurements. HPB (Oxford) 2015;17:471–476.
30 Haegele S, Reiter S, Wanek D, Offensperger F, Pereyra D, Stremitzer S, Fleischmann E, Brostjan C, Gruenberger T, Starlinger P: Perioperative non-invasive indocyanine green-clearance testing to predict postoperative outcome after liver resection. PLoS One 2016;11:e0165481.
31 Olmedilla L, Lisbona CJ, Perez-Pena JM, Lopez-Baena JA, Garutti I, Salcedo M, Sanz J, Tisner M, Asencio JM, Fernandez-Quero L, Banares R: Early measurement of indocyanine green clearance accurately predicts short-term outcomes after liver transplantation. Transplantation 2016;100:613–620.
32 Takasaki T, Kobayashi S, Suzuki S, Muto H, Marada M, Yamana Y, Nagaoka T: Predetermining postoperative hepatic function for hepatectomies. Int Surg 1980;65:309–313.
33 Fujio N, Sakai K, Kinoshita H, Hirohashi K, Kubo S, Iwasa R, Lee KC: Results of treatment of patients with hepatocellular carcinoma with severe cirrhosis of the liver. World J Surg 1989;13:211–217; discussion 217–218.
34 Hemming AW, Scudamore CH, Shackleton CR, Pudek M, Erb SR: Indocyanine green clearance as a predictor of successful hepatic resection in cirrhotic patients. Am J Surg 1992;163:515–518.
35 Miyagawa S, Makuuchi M, Kawasaki S, Kakazu T: Criteria for safe hepatic resection. Am J Surg 1995;169:589–594.
36 Fan ST, Lai EC, Lo CM, Ng IO, Wong J: Hospital mortality of major hepatectomy for hepatocellular carcinoma associated with cirrhosis. Arch Surg 1995;130:198–203.
37 Wu CC, Ho WL, Yeh DC, Huang CR, Liu TJ, P'Eng FK: Hepatic resection of hepatocellular carcinoma in cirrhotic livers: is it unjustified in impaired liver function? Surgery 1996;120:34–39.
38 Lau H, Man K, Fan ST, Yu WC, Lo CM, Wong J: Evaluation of preoperative hepatic function in patients with hepatocellular carcinoma undergoing hepatectomy. Br J Surg 1997;84:1255–1259.
39 Makuuchi M, Kosuge T, Takayama T, Yamazaki S, Kakazu T, Miyagawa S, Kawasaki S: Surgery for small liver cancers. Semin Surg Oncol 1993;9:298–304.
40 Imamura H, Sano K, Sugawara Y, Kokudo N, Makuuchi M: Assessment of hepatic reserve for indication of hepatic resection: decision tree incorporating indocyanine green test. J Hepatobiliary Pancreat Surg 2005;12:16–22.
41 Makuuchi M, Kokudo N, Arii S, Futagawa S, Kaneko S, Kawasaki S, Matsuyama Y, Okazaki M, Okita K, Omata M, Saida Y, Takayama T, Yamaoka Y: Development of evidence-based clinical guidelines for the diagnosis and treatment of hepatocellular carcinoma in Japan. Hepatol Res 2008;38:37–51.
42 Sakka SG, Reinhart K, Meier-Hellmann A: Prognostic value of the indocyanine green plasma disappearance rate in critically ill patients. Chest 2002;122:1715–1720.
43 Merle U, Sieg O, Stremmel W, Encke J, Eisenbach C: Sensitivity and specificity of plasma disappearance rate of indocyanine green as a prognostic indicator in acute liver failure. BMC Gastroenterol 2009;9:91.
44 Zoller B, Spanaus K, Gerster R, Fasshauer M, Stehberger PA, Klinzing S, Vergopoulos A, von Eckardstein A, Bechir M: ICG-liver test versus new biomarkers as prognostic markers for prolonged length of stay in critically ill patients – a prospective study of accuracy for prediction of length of stay in the ICU. Ann Intensive Care 2014;4:19.
45 Horvatits T, Kneidinger N, Drolz A, Roedl K, Rutter K, Kluge S, Trauner M, Fuhrmann V: Prognostic impact of ICG-PDR in patients with hypoxic hepatitis. Ann Intensive Care 2015;5:47.
46 Yamamoto Y, Ikai I, Kume M, Sakai Y, Yamauchi A, Shinohara H, Morimoto T, Shimahara Y, Yamamoto M, Yamaoka Y: New simple technique for hepatic parenchymal resection using a Cavitron Ultrasonic Surgical Aspirator and bipolar cautery equipped with a channel for water dripping. World J Surg 1999;23:1032–1037.
47 Nagino M, Kamiya J, Nishio H, Ebata T, Arai T, Nimura Y: Two hundred forty consecutive portal vein embolizations before extended hepatectomy for biliary cancer: surgical outcome and long-term follow-up. Ann Surg 2006;243:364–372.
48 Yokoyama Y, Nishio H, Ebata T, Igami T, Sugawara G, Nagino M: Value of indocyanine green clearance of the future liver remnant in predicting outcome after resection for biliary cancer. Br J Surg 2010;97:1260–1268.
49 Yokoyama Y, Ebata T, Igami T, Sugawara G, Mizuno T, Yamaguchi J, Nagino M: The predictive value of indocyanine green clearance in future liver remnant for posthepatectomy liver failure following hepatectomy with extrahepatic bile duct resection. World J Surg 2016;40:1440–1447.
50 Ohwada S, Kawate S, Hamada K, Yamada T, Sunose Y, Tsutsumi H, Tago K, Okabe T: Perioperative real-time monitoring of indocyanine green clearance by pulse spectrophotometry predicts remnant liver functional reserve in resection of hepatocellular carcinoma. Br J Surg 2006;93:339–346.
51 Lau L, Christophi C, Nikfarjam M, Starkey G, Goodwin M, Weinberg L, Ho L, Muralidharan V: Assessment of liver remnant using ICG clearance intraoperatively during vascular exclusion: early experience with the ALIIVE technique. HPB Surg 2015;2015:757052.
52 De Liguori Carino N, O'Reilly DA, Dajani K, Ghaneh P, Poston GJ, Wu AV: Perioperative use of the LiMON method of indocyanine green elimination measurement for the prediction and early detection of post-hepatectomy liver failure. Eur J Surg Oncol 2009;35:957–962.

53 Hori T, Iida T, Yagi S, Taniguchi K, Yamamoto C, Mizuno S, Yamagiwa K, Isaji S, Uemoto S: $K_{(ICG)}$ value, a reliable real-time estimator of graft function, accurately predicts outcomes in adult living-donor liver transplantation. Liver Transpl 2006;12:605–613.
54 Levesque E, Saliba F, Benhamida S, Ichai P, Azoulay D, Adam R, Castaing D, Samuel D: Plasma disappearance rate of indocyanine green: a tool to evaluate early graft outcome after liver transplantation. Liver Transpl 2009;15:1358–1364.
55 Schneider L, Spiegel M, Latanowicz S, Weigand MA, Schmidt J, Werner J, Stremmel W, Eisenbach C: Noninvasive indocyanine green plasma disappearance rate predicts early complications, graft failure or death after liver transplantation. Hepatobiliary Pancreat Dis Int 2011;10:362–368.
56 De Graaf W, Hausler S, Heger M, van Ginhoven TM, van Cappellen G, Bennink RJ, Kullak-Ublick GA, Hesselmann R, van Gulik TM, Stieger B: Transporters involved in the hepatic uptake of (99m)Tc-mebrofenin and indocyanine green. J Hepatol 2011;54:738–745.
57 Stockmann M, Lock JF, Riecke B, Heyne K, Martus P, Fricke M, Lehmann S, Niehues SM, Schwabe M, Lemke AJ, Neuhaus P: Prediction of postoperative outcome after hepatectomy with a new bedside test for maximal liver function capacity. Ann Surg 2009;250:119–125.
58 Lock JF, Schwabauer E, Martus P, Videv N, Pratschke J, Malinowski M, Neuhaus P, Stockmann M: Early diagnosis of primary nonfunction and indication for reoperation after liver transplantation. Liver Transpl 2010;16:172–180.
59 Namihisa T, Nambu M, Kobayashi N, Kuroda H: The constitutional indocyanine green excretory defect – report of four cases. Gastroenterol Jpn 1975;10:70–76.
60 Ashwell G, Morell AG: The role of surface carbohydrates in the hepatic recognition and transport of circulating glycoproteins. Adv Enzymol Relat Areas Mol Biol 1974;41:99–128.
61 Vera DR, Krohn KA, Stadalnik RC, Scheibe PO: Tc-99m galactosyl-neoglycoalbumin: in vitro characterization of receptor-mediated binding. J Nucl Med 1984;25:779–787.
62 Vera DR, Krohn KA, Stadalnik RC, Scheibe PO: Tc-99m-galactosyl-neoglycoalbumin: in vivo characterization of receptor-mediated binding to hepatocytes. Radiology 1984;151:191–196.
63 Vera DR, Stadalnik RC, Krohn KA: Technetium-99m galactosyl-neoglycoalbumin: preparation and preclinical studies. J Nucl Med 1985;26:1157–1167.
64 Sawamura T, Nakada H, Hazama H, Shiozaki Y, Sameshima Y, Tashiro Y: Hyperasialoglycoproteinemia in patients with chronic liver diseases and/or liver cell carcinoma. Asialoglycoprotein receptor in cirrhosis and liver cell carcinoma. Gastroenterology 1984;87:1217–1221.
65 Kudo M, Todo A, Ikekubo K, Hino M, Yonekura Y, Yamamoto K, Torizuka K: Functional hepatic imaging with receptor-binding radiopharmaceutical: clinical potential as a measure of functioning hepatocyte mass. Gastroenterol Jpn 1991;26:734–741.
66 Ha-Kawa SK, Tanaka Y: A quantitative model of technetium-99m-DTPA-galactosyl-HSA for the assessment of hepatic blood flow and hepatic binding receptor. J Nucl Med 1991;32:2233–2240.
67 Koizumi K, Uchiyama G, Arai T, Ainoda T, Yoda Y: A new liver functional study using Tc-99m DTPA-galactosyl human serum albumin: evaluation of the validity of several functional parameters. Ann Nucl Med 1992;6:83–87.
68 Kudo M, Todo A, Ikekubo K, Yamamoto K, Vera DR, Stadalnik RC: Quantitative assessment of hepatocellular function through in vivo radioreceptor imaging with technetium 99m galactosyl human serum albumin. Hepatology 1993;17:814–819.
69 Kubota Y, Kitagawa S, Inoue K, Ha-Kawa SK, Kojima M, Tanaka Y: Hepatic functional scintigraphic imaging with 99mtechnetium galactosyl serum albumin. Hepatogastroenterology 1993;40:32–36.
70 Kudo M, Todo A, Ikekubo K, Hino M: Receptor index via hepatic asialoglycoprotein receptor imaging: correlation with chronic hepatocellular damage. Am J Gastroenterol 1992;87:865–870.
71 Wu J, Ishikawa N, Takeda T, Tanaka Y, Pan XQ, Sato M, Todoroki T, Hatakeyama R, Itai Y: The functional hepatic volume assessed by 99mTc-GSA hepatic scintigraphy. Ann Nucl Med 1995;9:229–235.
72 Imaeda T, Kanematsu M, Asada S, Seki M, Doi H, Saji S: Utility of Tc-99m GSA SPECT imaging in estimation of functional volume of liver segments in health and liver diseases. Clin Nucl Med 1995;20:322–328.
73 Matsuzaki S, Onda M, Tajiri T, Kim DY: Hepatic lobar differences in progression of chronic liver disease: correlation of asialoglycoprotein scintigraphy and hepatic functional reserve. Hepatology 1997;25:828–832.
74 Sugai Y, Komatani A, Hosoya T, Yamaguchi K: Response to percutaneous transhepatic portal embolization: new proposed parameters by 99mTc-GSA SPECT and their usefulness in prognostic estimation after hepatectomy. J Nucl Med 2000;41:421–425.
75 Onodera Y, Takahashi K, Togashi T, Sugai Y, Tamaki N, Miyasaka K: Clinical assessment of hepatic functional reserve using 99mTc DTPA galactosyl human serum albumin SPECT to prognosticate chronic hepatic diseases – validation of the use of SPECT and a new indicator. Ann Nucl Med 2003;17:181–188.
76 Geisel D, Ludemann L, Hamm B, Denecke T: Imaging-based liver function tests – past, present and future. Rofo 2015;187:863–871.
77 Yoshida M, Shiraishi S, Sakaguchi F, Utsunomiya D, Tashiro K, Tomiguchi S, Okabe H, Beppu T, Baba H, Yamashita Y: A quantitative index measured on $^{99}$mTc GSA SPECT/CT 3D fused images to evaluate severe fibrosis in patients with chronic liver disease. Jpn J Radiol 2012;30:435–441.
78 Usui T, Kawamoto H: A new method for the estimation of blood indocyanine green with a decolorization reagent (Article in Japanese). Rinsho Byori 1970;18:882–884.
79 Mao Y, Du S, Ba J, Li F, Yang H, Lu X, Sang X, Li S, Che L, Tong J, Xu Y, Xu H, Zhao H, Chi T, Liu F, Du Y, Zhang X, Wang X, Dong J, Zhong S, Huang J, Yu Y, Wang J: Using dynamic 99mT c-GSA SPECT/CT fusion images for hepatectomy planning and postoperative liver failure prediction. Ann Surg Oncol 2015;22:1301–1307.
80 Iimuro Y, Kashiwagi T, Yamanaka J, Hirano T, Saito S, Sugimoto T, Watanabe S, Kuroda N, Okada T, Asano Y, Uyama N, Fujimoto J: Preoperative estimation of asialoglycoprotein receptor expression in the remnant liver from CT/99mTc-GSA SPECT fusion images correlates well with postoperative liver function parameters. J Hepatobiliary Pancreat Sci 2010;17:673–681.
81 Akaki S, Mitsumori A, Kanazawa S, Togami I, Takeda Y, Hiraki Y: Lobar decrease in 99mTc-GSA accumulation in hilar cholangiocarcinoma. J Nucl Med 1999;40:394–398.
82 Sugahara K, Togashi H, Takahashi K, Onodera Y, Sanjo M, Misawa K, Suzuki A, Adachi T, Ito J, Okumoto K, Hattori E, Takeda T, Watanabe H, Saito K, Saito T, Sugai Y, Kawata S: Separate analysis of asialoglycoprotein receptors in the right and left hepatic lobes using Tc-GSA SPECT. Hepatology 2003;38:1401–1409.
83 Yumoto Y, Yagi T, Sato S, Nouso K, Kobayashi Y, Ohmoto M, Yumoto E, Nagaya I, Nakatsukasa H: Preoperative estimation of remnant hepatic function using fusion images obtained by $^{99m}$Tc-labelled galactosyl-human serum albumin liver scintigraphy and computed tomography. Br J Surg 2010;97:934–944.
84 Sumiyoshi T, Shima Y, Tokorodani R, Okabayashi T, Kozuki A, Hata Y, Noda Y, Murata Y, Nakamura T, Uka K: CT/99mTc-GSA SPECT fusion images demonstrate functional differences between the liver lobes. World J Gastroenterol 2013;19:3217–3225.
85 Sumiyoshi T, Shima Y, Okabayashi T, Kozuki A, Hata Y, Noda Y, Kouno M, Miyagawa K, Tokorodani R, Saisaka Y, Tokumaru T, Nakamura T, Morita S: Liver function assessment using 99mTc-GSA single-photon emission computed tomography (SPECT)/CT fusion imaging in hilar bile duct cancer: a retrospective study. Surgery 2016;160:118–126.
86 Tsuruga Y, Kamiyama T, Kamachi H, Shimada S, Wakayama K, Orimo T, Kakisaka T, Yokoo H, Taketomi A: Significance of functional hepatic resection rate calculated using 3D CT/$^{99m}$Tc-galactosyl human serum albumin single-photon emission computed tomography fusion imaging. World J Gastroenterol 2016;22:4373–4379.
87 Yoshida M, Shiraishi S, Sakaguchi F, Utsunomiya D, Tashiro K, Tomiguchi S, Okabe H, Beppu T, Baba H, Yamashita Y: Fused 99m-Tc-GSA SPECT/CT imaging for the preoperative evaluation of postoperative liver function: can the liver uptake index predict postoperative hepatic functional reserve? Jpn J Radiol 2012;30:255–262.
88 Kubo S, Shiomi S, Tanaka H, Shuto T, Takemura S, Mikami S, Uenishi T, Nishino Y, Hirohashi K, Kawamura E, Kinoshita H: Evaluation of the effect of portal vein embolization on liver function by $^{99m}$tc-galactosyl human serum albumin scintigraphy. J Surg Res 2002;107:113–118.
89 Sumiyoshi T, Shima Y, Okabayashi T, Noda Y, Hata Y, Murata Y, Kozuki A, Tokumaru T, Nakamura T, Uka K: Functional discrepancy between two liver lobes after hemilobe biliary drainage in patients with jaundice and bile duct cancer: an appraisal using $^{99m}$Tc-GSA SPECT/CT fusion imaging. Radiology 2014;273:444–451.
90 Bennink RJ, Dinant S, Erdogan D, Heijnen BH, Straatsburg IH, van Vliet AK, van Gulik TM: Preoperative assessment of postoperative remnant liver function using hepatobiliary scintigraphy. J Nucl Med 2004;45:965–971.
91 De Graaf W, van Lienden KP, Dinant S, Roelofs JJ, Busch OR, Gouma DJ, Bennink RJ, van Gulik TM: Assessment of future remnant liver function using hepatobiliary scintigraphy in patients undergoing major liver resection. J Gastrointest Surg 2010;14:369–378.
92 De Graaf W, van Lienden KP, van Gulik TM, Bennink RJ: $^{99m}$Tc-mebrofenin hepatobiliary scintigraphy with SPECT for the assessment of hepatic function and liver functional volume before partial hepatectomy. J Nucl Med 2010;51:229–236.
93 De Graaf W, van Lienden KP, van den Esschert JW, Bennink RJ, van Gulik TM: Increase in future remnant liver function after preoperative portal vein embolization. Br J Surg 2011;98:825–834.
94 Cieslak KP, Huisman F, Bais T, Bennink RJ, van Lienden KP, Verheij J, Besselink MG, Busch ORC, van Gulik TM: Future remnant liver function as predictive factor for the hypertrophy response after portal vein embolization. Surgery 2017;162:37–47.
95 Bae KE, Kim SY, Lee SS, Kim KW, Won HJ, Shin YM, Kim PN, Lee MG: Assessment of hepatic function with Gd-EOB-DTPA-enhanced hepatic MRI. Dig Dis 2012;30:617–622.

Visceral Medicine

Original Article

Visc Med 2017;33:456–461
DOI: 10.1159/000479476

Published online: November 30, 2017

# Did the International ALPPS Meeting 2015 Have an Impact on Daily Practice? The Hamburg Barmbek Experience of 58 Cases

Gregor A. Stavrou[a, b] Marcello Donati[a, c] Mohammad H. Fard-Aghaie[a] Martin Zeile[b, d] Tessa M. Huber[a] Axel Stang[b, e] Karl J. Oldhafer[a, b]

[a] General and Visceral Surgery, Surgical Oncology, Asklepios Hospital Barmbek, Hamburg, Germany;
[b] Semmelweis Medical Faculty, Campus Hamburg, Hamburg, Germany;
[c] Department of Surgery, Vittorio-Emanuele University Hospital Catania, Catania, Italy;
[d] Diagnostic and Interventional Radiology, Asklepios Hospital Barmbek, Hamburg, Germany;
[e] Medical Oncology, Asklepios Hospital Barmbek, Hamburg, Germany

**Keywords**
ALPPS · In-situ split · Liver · Two-stage

**Summary**
**Background:** ALPPS (associating liver partition and portal vein ligation for staged hepatectomy) was introduced only 10 years ago and has gained wide acceptance as a variation of staged procedures in liver surgery. It has been criticized for its high morbidity and mortality, which all centers reported in their initial series. **Methods:** After a world expert meeting in Hamburg in 2015 where all experts in the field met to discuss this method, caveats were extracted and formulated. We researched our complete prospective ALPPS database to see if the recommendations had any impact on outcome. **Results:** In total, we performed 58 ALPPS procedures in our center. 33 patients were operated on before, 25 after the meeting. Results in terms of morbidity and mortality were significantly better after the meeting, as were patient selection and strategy. **Conclusion:** In our own center's experience, the implementation of the meetings' recommendations and the information gathered through this valuable exchange had a dramatic impact on results. Having performed 58 ALPPS procedures in total, we can now conclude that ALPPS has become much safer in our hands since the 2015 meeting and that morbidity and mortality are no longer the issue to be discussed. Future research must focus on oncologic outcomes in these patients.



## Introduction

The first in-situ split procedure performed by Hans Schlitt in Regensburg in 2007 was adopted 10 years later as a new method to face extensive liver disease requiring staged procedures by many centers in Germany and worldwide [1–13].

After the first German multi-institutional series was published in 2012 [3], the HPB (hepato-pancreato-biliary surgery) community was excited, fascinated, and yet somewhat shocked by the high morbidity and mortality (M&M) that the new method – today referred to as ALPPS (associating liver partition and portal vein ligation for staged hepatectomy) [14] – had shown to produce. Many in the conservative arm of the HPB community advocated the immediate stop of the use of this procedure [8, 15–22]; however, others realized the potential of the new strategy once HPB surgeons had overcome the initial learning curve, and proposed a unique approach to this newly introduced method with the founding of the international ALPPS registry (*www.alpps.net*). With this, a platform was given to all to study actual results and to learn and further develop the method. With all the known flaws and limitations of such registries, it still remains a unique dataset. At the time when laparoscopic cholecystectomy was introduced, no one had thought of setting up a registry. Even laparoscopic bowel or liver surgery was started without monitoring; registries were implemented 10 years after the use of these techniques had become widespread. The ALPPS registry has been extensively studied and has produced helpful results so far including the understanding of pitfalls [23–26].

In February 2015, an International Expert Meeting on ALPPS took place in Hamburg (*www.alpps.co*), bringing together all

KARGER

Fax +49 761 4 52 07 14
Information@Karger.com
www.karger.com



Accessible online at:
www.karger.com/vis

Dr. med. Dr. habil. Gregor A. Stavrou
Klinik für Allgemein- und Viszeralchirurgie, Chirurgische Onkologie
Asklepios Klinik Barmbek
Rübenkamp 220, 22291 Hamburg, Germany
g.stavrou@asklepios.com

known experts in this field as well as prominent critics to discuss all aspects of the procedure over 2 days. The aim of the meeting was to reach a consensus on how the procedure could be advanced according to key recommendations of the meeting [27]. The involvement of our center with ALPPS started in 2011 [28] after a personal communication with Hans Schlitt. The purpose of this study is to show our experience over 6 years divided into a pre- and post-meeting period. With 58 ALPPS procedures performed in total, this appears to be one of the largest series worldwide.

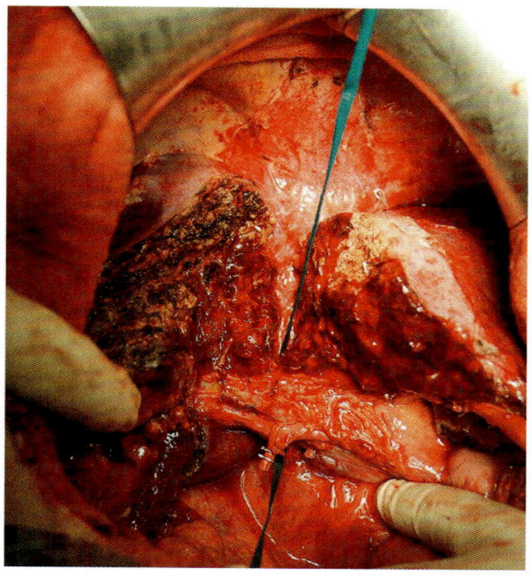

**Fig. 1.** Intraoperative photograph of an ALPPS step 1 from the early era. Performed as a full parenchymal transection down to the vena cava using the anterior approach with a liver hanging maneuver as well as adding Launois' maneuver and tagging of anatomical structures (red tag around right hepatic artery).

## Methods

Using our institution's prospective database for all ALPPS cases, we performed a complete workup of all patient data. We divided the identified 58 patients into 2 subgroups – before and after the 2015 ALPPS Meeting in Hamburg. We then analyzed technique, outcome, morbidity, and mortality, and provided follow-up for the first group.

From 03/2011 to 03/2017, 1,016 liver resections were performed in our department. A hypertrophy concept for staged procedures was used in 136 patients (3 classic 2-stage hepatectomies with portal vein ligation, 75 portal vein embolizations (PVE), 58 ALPPS), representing 13% of our total collective. As for colorectal liver metastases (CRLM), it is important to mention that all our patients received four cycles (more in a few cases) of modern chemotherapy (FOLFOX/FOLFIRI or later FOLFOXIRI) combined with antibodies (cetuximab/bevacizumab) to gain systemic control upfront, and also that stable disease or partial remission was a selection criterion for eligibility for an ALPPS approach.

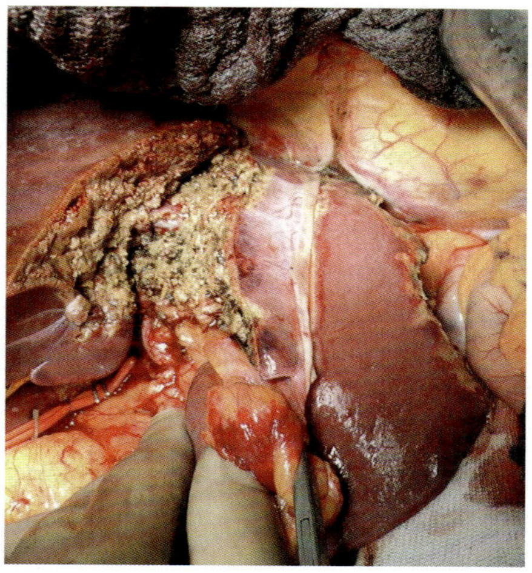

**Fig. 2.** Intraoperative photograph of an ALPPS step 1 from the post-meeting period. Performed as a partial (50%) parenchymal transection down to the level of the middle hepatic vein and tagging of anatomical structures (red tag around right hepatic artery).

## Results

*ALPPS 03/2011 to 02/2015 (Pre-Meeting Period)*

A total of 33 ALPPS procedures were performed in this first period. Indications varied. ALPPS was mainly performed for CRLM (n = 22). Bilobar disease was present in 12 cases. A 'liver first approach' was used in 2 patients. Non-CRLM indications (n = 11) were hepatocellular carcinoma (HCC), cholangiocellular carcinoma (CCC), gastrointestinal stromal tumor, and other metastases. Mean age was 66.6 years with a mean Charlson comorbidity index of 9. 5 patients underwent ALPPS after PVE failed to induce hypertrophy ('rescue ALPPS'). Mean standardized future liver remnant (sFLR) volumes were 20% before step 1 (volume of additional atypical resections in the FLR was not measured) and 34% before step 2, with an absolute mean growth of 79%. In this period, we had already adopted a longer interval between steps, resulting in a mean period of 22 days.

Resections finally completed resulted in right hepatectomy plus multiple atypical resections in the FLR in 2 cases, extended right hepatectomy in 19 cases, and extended right hepatectomy plus atypical resections in the FLR in 10 cases. During step 1, we performed full transection with a liver hanging maneuver in the anterior approach and taping of structures as previously reported [29] (fig. 1); in 3 patients, a partial ALPPS procedure was performed.

Of the 33 patients, 31 entered into step 2, while 2 patients died after step 1 (a 78-year-old gentleman with CCC suffered cardiac failure on postoperative day (POD) 2 and could not be resuscitated; the other 73-year-old gentleman with HCC and nutritive-toxic Child A cirrhosis developed acute chronic liver failure as well as consecutive multiple organ failure after step 1 and died). No other patients manifested severe complications after step 1. Patients going on to step 2 suffered complications greater than Clavien-Dindo Grade IIIa in 27%. 5 patients were lost after step 2, accounting for an overall mortality of 20 and 15%, respectively, after completion of both steps.

The 5 patients lost after step 2 suffered liver failure. In 3 patients, the cause of liver failure was a small-for-size syndrome: 1 patient had a pre-step 2 sFLR of 22%, another patient had transient liver failure according to the International Study Group of Liver Surgery (ISGLS) definition [30] with a bilirubin level of 2.2 mg/dl pre-step 2; the third patient likely had a general problem with liver regeneration because his liver failed to show a hypertrophic response in spite of a technically good PVE with the sFLR only growing to 25.5% even after ALPPS step 1. The other 2 patients presented with liver failure provoked by cholestasis and cholangitis: Unfortunately, in 1 patient with gallbladder carcinoma, FLR volumetry was inappropriately performed and his sFLR was later corrected to be 19%. The other patient suffered septic multiple organ failure. He had undergone ALPPS as a rescue procedure for CRLM.

After a 4-month stay in the intensive care unit due to severe aspiration pneumonia following resection of a stenosing sigmoid primary cancer, he refused chemotherapy, and surgery was left as the only option for his liver metastases. Even though the liver remnant had shown good hypertrophy, the patient was in severely impaired general condition and developed cholangitis and liver failure after step 2.

At this time, there were no restrictions for the use of ALPPS, although it was not performed for Klatskin tumors. Comorbidities and age were not seen as criteria based on which a patient considered fit for conventional liver resection would have been denied the procedure. Volumetry of the liver remnant was introduced in that period, but it was not standardized and had technical difficulties and sometimes produced suboptimal results. ALPPS procedures were performed by the same 3 surgeons with hepatobiliary specialist training.

*ALPPS 03/2015 to 03/2017 (Post-Meeting Period)*

A total of 25 ALPPS procedures were performed in the post-meeting period. This does not resemble an increase in the use of the ALPPS concept since the total number of liver resections/year increased to over 200 in this era. CRLM was the main indication for ALPPS in the majority of cases (n = 19). In 6 selected patients, other indications were approved (liver metastases from neuroendocrine tumor, solitary fibrous tumor of hemangiopericytoma type, duodenal cancer, CCC, 2 Klatskin tumors). All patients with CRLM suffered bilobar disease, therefore a 'liver first approach' was utilized more often with 9 cases in total [31]. With 52.6 years, the mean age was significantly lower, as was the Charlson comorbidity index at 7.

Mean sFLR volumes were 19.75% before step 1 (volume of additional atypical resections in the FLR was not measured) and 30.58% before step 2, with an absolute mean growth of 59%. Again, the interval between steps was longer at 24 days. Resections finally completed resulted in right hepatectomy plus multiple atypical resections in the FLR in 1 patient, extended right hepatectomy in 5 patients, and extended right hepatectomy plus atypical resections in the FRL in 14 patients. 1 monosegment 7 reverse ALPPS was included. In this period, during step 1, we performed partial (50%) liver transection with preservation of the middle hepatic vein and without mobilizing the right liver in 20 patients (fig. 2). Hybrid ALPPS – a combination of parenchymal transection of 50% with tumor clearance in the FLR and a right PVE 1 week later – was done in 3 patients; only in 1 patient we managed to go on to step 2. In 2 patients with Klatskin tumors, right + segment 4 PVE was followed by laparoscopic parenchymal transection as a rescue procedure for insufficient FLR growth.

Of the 25 patients, only 21 went on to step 2. Reasons for drop-out (16%) were slow hypertrophy and rapid progress of disease while waiting for step 2 in 2 patients. Of the remaining 2 patients, 1 patient with insufficient hypertrophy after hybrid ALPPS received a 'rescue' right hepatic vein embolization (HVE) after waiting for months; and the other patient with Klatskin tumor, who had undergone laparoscopic hybrid partial ALPPS as step 1, repeatedly refused to go on to step 2 despite good hypertrophy because his clinical condition was excellent and cholestasis was well controlled. Overall, severe morbidity defined as greater than Clavien-Dindo Grade IIIa occurred significantly less with 16%. We did not lose any patient directly due to ALPPS; however, 1 patient who failed to demonstrate hypertrophy of the FLR after step 1 underwent 'rescue PVE' of a newly developed segment 4 portal collateral followed by 'rescue right HVE', which eventually produced adequate hypertrophy. He was able to undergo right trisectionectomy 4 months after step 1; however, he developed an unexplained 40 °C fever and died of septic multiple organ failure on POD 14. Hence the accurate overall mortality was 4% in the post-meeting period. Results are summarized in table 1.

## Discussion

Is an expert meeting able to have an impact on the daily routine and practice of a new method? If IDEAL (Idea, Development, Exploration, Assessment, Long-term Follow-up) guidelines [32] on how to reach a formal consensus on a new method are explored, probably not. Still, this expert meeting on ALPPS can be considered extraordinary because it fostered discussions between leaders in the field and gave way to new variations, insights, and experiences across the world. It also included all prominent voices expressing their concerns about the use of this method, cautioning the community to realize the need for some change to enable better results. The meeting's extracts were published in *Annals of Surgery* in 2016 [27].

Taking on board what we learned in the ALPPS meeting, we aimed for a better selection of patients. This is reflected in the fact that patients treated after the meeting were significantly younger and had less comorbidities. Meticulous planning of the operation based on diagnostic imaging is important as well as an interest and expertise in volumetry for calculating the sFLR [33–36]. This was implemented in our center in a way that only 1 radiologist with a special interest in HPB radiology, who also performed PVE himself, was in charge of volumetric analysis. From a technical point of view, we opted for a decrease in trauma during step 1 as proposed by de Santibañes et al. [37] and adopted partial ALPPS aiming at 50% parenchymal transection with preservation of the middle hepatic vein. Derived from the principle of formation of new portal collaterals as an obstacle in the progress towards hypertrophy in our PVE patients [38], we deliberately took time during step 1 to ensure the division of all possible segment 4 portal collaterals coming from the left portal branches as identified by intraoperative ultrasound. The preparation in the hepatoduodenal ligament was minimized to a direct access to the portal vein for its transection as well as tagging of the right hepatic artery. Before the ALPPS meeting, we used the liver hanging maneuver and anterior approach in step1; now hanging is no longer used. However, we still avoid mobilization of the right liver during step 1.

Looking at our data, we can conclude that we succeeded in enabling sufficient growth in the FLR to go on to step 2 in most pa-

**Table 1.** Summary of patient characteristics and data about the ALPPS collective in both the pre- and post-meeting period

| | Before meeting (n = 33) | After meeting (n = 25) |
|---|---|---|
| Mean age, years | 66.6 | 52.6 |
| Charlson comorbidity index, n | 9 | 7 |
| Colorectal liver metastases, n | | |
| No | 11 | 6 |
| Yes | 22 | 19 |
| Bilobar, n | 12 | 19 |
| Liver first, n | 2 | 9 |
| Right hepatectomy (RH) + atypical resection S2/3, n | 2 | 1 |
| Extended right hemihepatectomy, n | 19 | 5 |
| Extended RH + atypical resection S2/3, n | 10 | 14 |
| Monosegment ALPPS, n | 0 | 1 |
| Partial ALPPS, n | 3 | 25 |
| No mobilization technique, n | 2 | 20 |
| Hybrid ALPPS, n | 0 | 5 |
| Step 1 only, n | 2 | 4 |
| Dropout before Step 2, n | 2 | 4 |
| Reason for dropout | 2 deaths | 2 progress<br>1 rescue hepatic vein embolization (HVE),<br>1 patient refused step 2 |
| Morbidity > IIIa, % | 27 | 16 |
| Mortality, % | 20 overall<br>15 in completed ALPPS | 4 overall<br>n = 1 lost after HVE (4 months after step 2) |
| Standardized future liver remnant (sFLR) before Step 1 (mean), additional resections in FLR not measured, % | 20 | 19.75 |
| sFLR before Step 2 (mean), % | 34 | 30.5 |
| Hypertrophy, % | 79 | 59 |
| Interval Step 1/2 (mean), n | 22 | 24 |

tients. Giving that the starting sFRL was equivalent in the 2 groups (below 20%) before step 1, patients did not experience the same amount of growth with partial ALPPS (79 vs. 59%) in their FLR; nevertheless, there was enough volume to go on to step 2. The effectiveness of partial ALPPS was also studied multi-institutionally with the results leading to the same conclusion [39].

Gaining systemic control of the tumor upfront in patients with CRLM seems logical in these borderline resectable cases. Stable disease or partial remission seems a good criterion to select patients eligible for an ALPPS approach. We have not seen any impairment in hypertrophy even in partial ALPPS after chemotherapy, which corroborates the published data [40]. Hence we believe that 3–4 cycles of neoadjuvant chemotherapy are adequate prior to surgery, allowing good tumor control without impairing liver regeneration.

From the beginning, it was our policy to not strictly follow the '9-day' dogma between the 2 steps, and this has not changed in the post-meeting period. However, with a cautious view on liver function assessment, we now wait slightly longer before step 2 to ensure normal liver function – lessons learned from the ALPPS meeting and from experiences published by the registry [24, 41]. From current data based on all kinds of liver function assessment tests (e.g. HIDA scan), we now know that volume does not immediately equal function [42, 43]; hence we have learned to be cautious in that regard. It could be argued that a 3-week waiting time between steps for patients with CRLM comes close to the waiting period after PVE [20, 44]. However, this is not really the point; our patients with CRLM all suffered bilobar disease and had pre-step 1 sFLRs of far below 20%. Even with a perfect result after PVE, it would be unlikely that a patient could go on to step 2 after 3 weeks.

Undoubtedly, step 2 surgery after partial ALPPS is technically much more challenging compared to step 2 after full ALPPS, especially after a longer waiting period. For this reason, we adhere to the principle of the same 2 surgeons with experience in ALPPS being in charge in the operating theatre for both step 1 and 2, with an independent assessment of the anatomy being carried out by each surgeon before transection of structures. Where Launois' maneuver is feasible, it enables transection far away from the left hilar structures with a stapler device, which has proven to be a good method in our practice. Our experience with hybrid ALPPS [45] has been inconclusive so far. We opted for this method in CRLM patients requiring extensive resection of metastases in the FLR in whom we felt portal occlusion would be too invasive at this point.

Of 3 patients with CRLM undergoing this procedure, 2 could not proceed to step 2 because of insufficient hypertrophy and disease progression. To accept a dropout rate of 4/25 patients with respect to their individual regenerative capacity of the liver was a new aspect for us in the post-meeting period. Still, a dropout rate of 16% is half that reported for PVE cases. On the other hand, we have found a new concept for the treatment of Klatskin tumors, as we still see ALPPS as an option in selected cases [46]. In 2 Klatskin tumor patients (Bismuth IIIa type), PVE extended to segment 4 was followed by laparoscopic partial ALPPS because hypertrophy of the sFLR was insufficient. After this, both patients had sufficient hypertrophy to go on to step 2. 1 patient refused step 2 surgery while the other received R0 clearance of his tumor without any complications. Next to the initially reported 'rescue ALPPS' after PVE failure [5], with advances in interventional technique and center experience, we can now also provide 'rescue PVE' for some new portal collaterals that form after step 1 as well as 'rescue HVE' if the FLR volume does not increase enough. We do not see PVE, 2-stage hepatectomy, and ALPPS as concurring methods for treating the same patients – they are rather variations of the same theme to treat selected patients who are at the far end of the resectability spectrum. Looking at this issue from the M&M perspective, ALPPS has proven to produce good results while maintaining an M&M comparable to large PVE series. The 5–6% mortality rate after PVE or 2-stage hepatectomy [19, 21, 47], and also our 4% mortality rate of ALPPS in the new era, highlight the fact that we are treating patients suffering from extensive disease with palliative chemotherapy as the only other option. This is consistent with data from the ALPPS registry, where mortality was 8% in total and 5% in patients suffering from CRLM and being <60 years of age [26]. With these complex oncologic strategies and technically even more complex surgeries, it is unlikely that we will ever reach a 0% mortality rate [48]. In this respect, we have to keep in mind that even palliative chemotherapy has a 90-day mortality of 5.5% according to large series [49]. The community should therefore come together more frequently and share their experience within special meetings as was done for ALPPS to further develop clinical strategies.

Since we seem to have conquered the problem of M&M 10 years after the ALPPS procedure was first performed, one big question remains: Does our strategy make sense oncologically? Our group was the first to advise caution on this issue after early recurrences were noted [50]. Still, if patients go through tumor clearance of the liver once, they have better survival, which we know from multiple series. And this is also true for patients treated with ALPPS [51, 52]. The difference is that with ALPPS disease-free survival may be lower than with conventional 2-stage hepatectomy, but survival maybe comparable [53, 54]. With all the advances in modern combination chemotherapy, it looks like survival on chemotherapy for CRLM is just reaching over 20 months in selected groups of patients [55, 56], but these data are very complex and include patients who successfully underwent surgery after chemotherapy. We know that patients after ALPPS can live longer than those not receiving ALPPS [52, 54], and survival data from larger series are to be awaited. However, unfortunately, there is currently no study comparing surgical approaches ad extremis with palliative chemotherapy in a prospective way.

## Conclusion

From our single center experience of 58 cases (33 pre- and 25 post-meeting), we can conclude that the Hamburg international ALPPS meeting had a tremendous impact on our practice of ALPPS. We have succeeded in reducing severe complications to 16% and have not lost any patients within 90 days of step 1 or 2. From a technical point of view, we have managed to implement partial ALPPS as an effective alternative that is equally effective in producing the required hypertrophy. The results achieved with partial ALPPS may not be exactly the same compared to complete ALPPS but are enough to proceed to the step 2 operation.

M&M should no longer be the main focus of discussion in ALPPS. To answer the question of oncologic benefit for the patients, we propose a randomized trial in patients with bilobar CRLM, with randomization to palliative chemotherapy alone or to staged surgical procedures including ALPPS after induction chemotherapy.

## Disclosure Statement

The authors declare no conflict of interest.

## References


1 Baumgart J, Lang S, Lang H: A new method for induction of liver hypertrophy prior to right trisectionectomy: a report of three cases. HPB (Oxford) 2011;13:71–72.
2 Lang SA, Loss M, Schlitt HJ: 'In-situ split' (ISS) liver resection: new aspects of technique and indication (Article in German). Zentralbl Chir 2014;139:212–129.
3 Schnitzbauer AA, Lang SA, Goessmann H, et al: Right portal vein ligation combined with in situ splitting induces rapid left lateral liver lobe hypertrophy enabling 2-staged extended right hepatic resection in small-for-size settings. Ann Surg 2012;255:405–414.
4 Hahn O, Dudás I, Pajor P, et al: ALPPS (associated liver partition and portal vein ligation for staged hepatectomy) – faster and more significant liver hypertrophy (Article in Hungarian). Magy Seb 2013;66:21–26.
5 Knoefel WT, Gabor I, Rehders A, et al: In situ liver transection with portal vein ligation for rapid growth of the future liver remnant in two-stage liver resection. Br J Surg 2013;100:388–394.
6 Li J, Girotti P, Königsrainer I, Ladurner R, Königsrainer A, Nadalin S: ALPPS in right trisectionectomy: a safe procedure to avoid postoperative liver failure? J Gastrointest Surg 2013;17:956–961.
7 Torres OJ, Fernandes Ede S, Oliveira CV, et al: Associating liver partition and portal vein ligation for staged hepatectomy (ALPPS): the Brazilian experience. Arq Bras Cir Dig 2013;26:40–43.
8 Dokmak S, Belghiti J: Which limits to the 'ALPPS' approach? Ann Surg 2012;256:e6, author reply e16–17.
9 Machado MAC, Makdissi FF, Surjan RC: Totally laparoscopic ALPPS is feasible and may be worthwhile. Ann Surg 2012;256:e13, author reply e16–19.
10 Sala S, Ardiles V, Ulla M, Alvarez F, Pekolj J, Santibañes E: Our initial experience with ALPPS technique: encouraging results. Updates Surg 2012;64:167–172.

11 Robles Campos R, Paricio PP, Conesa AL, Hernández CM, Pérez RG, Quiñonero MF: A new surgical strategy for multiple bilobular liver metastases: right portal occlusion and tourniquet in the parenchyma section line (Article in Spanish). Cir Esp 2012;90:191–196.
12 Guglielmi A, Ruzzenente A, Conci S, Valdegamberi A, Iacono C: How much remnant is enough in liver resection? Dig Surg 2012;29:6–17.
13 De Santibañes E, Alvarez FA, Ardiles V: How to avoid postoperative liver failure: a novel method. World J Surg 2011;36:125–128.
14 De Santibañes E, Clavien P-A: Playing Play-Doh to prevent postoperative liver failure: the 'ALPPS' approach. Ann Surg 2012;255:415–417.
15 Tanabe KK: Are we thinking? A commentary on 'Is partial-ALPPS safer than ALPPS? A single-center experience'. Ann Surg 2015;261:e93.
16 Tanabe KK: Commentary on 'Can we improve the morbidity and mortality associated with the associating liver partition with portal vein ligation for staged hepatectomy (ALPPS) procedure in the management of colorectal liver metastases?'. Commentary on ALPPS: march of progress. Surgery 2015;157:204–206.
17 Rohatgi S, Harrison EM, Powell JJ, Wigmore SJ: ALPPS: adverse outcomes demand clear justification in an era of improving survival for colorectal liver metastases. World J Surg 2014;39:1848–1849.
18 Figueras J, Belghiti J: The ALPPS approach: should we sacrifice basic therapeutic rules in the name of innovation? World J Surg 2014;38:1520–1521.
19 Kokudo N, Shindoh J: How can we safely climb the ALPPS? Updates Surg 2013;65:175–177.
20 Shindoh J, Vauthey J-N, Zimmitti G, et al: Analysis of the efficacy of portal vein embolization for patients with extensive liver malignancy and very low future liver remnant volume, including a comparison with the associating liver partition with portal vein ligation for staged hepatectomy approach. J Am Coll Surg 2013;217:126–133.
21 Aloia TA, Vauthey J-N: Associating liver partition and portal vein ligation for staged hepatectomy (ALPPS): what is gained and what is lost? Ann Surg 2012;256:e9, author reply e16–19.
22 Narita M, Oussoultzoglou E, Fuchshuber P, et al: What is a safe future liver remnant size in patients undergoing major hepatectomy for colorectal liver metastases and treated by intensive preoperative chemotherapy? Ann Surg Oncol 2012;19:2526–2538.
23 Buac S, Schadde E, Schnitzbauer AA, Vogt K, Hernandez-Alejandro R: The many faces of ALPPS: surgical indications and techniques among surgeons collaborating in the international registry. HPB (Oxford) 2016;18:442–448.
24 Schadde E, Raptis DA, Schnitzbauer AA, et al: Prediction of mortality after ALPPS stage-1: an analysis of 320 patients from the International ALPPS Registry. Ann Surg 2015;262:780–786.
25 Ratti F, Schadde E, Masetti M, et al: Strategies to increase the resectability of patients with colorectal liver metastases: a multi-center case-match analysis of ALPPS and conventional two-stage hepatectomy. Ann Surg Oncol 2015;22:1933–1942.
26 Schadde E, Ardiles V, Robles Campos R, et al: Early survival and safety of ALPPS: first report of the International ALPPS Registry. Ann Surg 2014;260:829–836, discussion 836–838.
27 Oldhafer KJ, Stavrou GA, van Gulik TM: ALPPS – where do we stand, where do we go? Eight recommendations from the first International Expert Meeting. Ann Surg 2016;263:839–841.
28 Donati M, Stavrou GA, Basile F, Gruttadauria S, Niehaus KJ, Oldhafer KJ: Combination of in situ split and portal ligation: lights and shadows of a new surgical procedure. Ann Surg 2012;256:e11–12, author reply e16–19.
29 Stavrou GA, Donati M, Niehaus KJ, et al: In-Situ-Split der Leber kombiniert mit Pfortaderligatur. Ein neuer Ansatz um die Resektabilität bei kolorektalen Lebermetastasen zu steigern. Z Gastroenterol 2012;50:K376.
30 Rahbari NN, Garden OJ, Padbury R, et al: Posthepatectomy liver failure: a definition and grading by the International Study Group of Liver Surgery (ISGLS). Surgery 2011;149:713–724.
31 Donati M, Stavrou GA, Stang A, Basile F, Oldhafer KJ: 'Liver-first' approach with ALPPS: the natural combination of two new concepts in liver surgery. Surg Oncol 2016;25:278–280.
32 McCulloch P, Altman DG, Campbell WB, et al: No surgical innovation without evaluation: the IDEAL recommendations. Lancet 2009;374:1105–1112.
33 Truant S, Boleslawski E, Sergent G, et al: Liver function following extended hepatectomy can be accurately predicted using remnant liver volume to body weight ratio. World J Surg 2015;39:1139–1201.
34 Truant S, Oberlin O, Sergent G, et al: Remnant liver volume to body weight ratio ≥0.5%: a new cut-off to estimate postoperative risks after extended resection in noncirrhotic liver. J Am Coll Surg 2007;204:22–33.
35 Vauthey JN, Chaoui A, Do KA, et al: Standardized measurement of the future liver remnant prior to extended liver resection: methodology and clinical associations. Surgery 2000;127:512–519.
36 Vauthey J-N, Abdalla EK, Doherty DA, et al: Body surface area and body weight predict total liver volume in Western adults. Liver Transpl 2002;8:233–240.
37 De Santibañes E, Alvarez FA, Ardiles V, Pekolj J, de Santibañes M: Inverting the ALPPS paradigm by minimizing first stage impact: the Mini-ALPPS technique. Langenbecks Arch Surg 2016;401:557–563.
38 Zeile M, Bakal A, Volkmer JE, et al: Identification of cofactors influencing hypertrophy of the future liver remnant after portal vein embolization – the effect of porto-portal collaterals on the embolized liver volume. Br J Radiol 2016;89:20160306.
39 Linecker M, Kambakamba P, Reiner CS, et al: How much liver needs to be transected in ALPPS? A translational study investigating the concept of less invasiveness. Surgery 2017;161:453–464.
40 Hasselgren K, Malagó M, Vyas S, et al: Neoadjuvant chemotherapy does not affect future liver remnant growth and outcomes of associating liver partition and portal vein ligation for staged hepatectomy. Surgery 2017;161:1255–1265.
41 Linecker M, Stavrou GA, Oldhafer KJ, et al: The ALPPS risk score: avoiding futile use of ALPPS. Ann Surg 2016;264:763–771.
42 Sparrelid E, Jonas E, Tzortzakakis A, et al: Dynamic evaluation of liver volume and function in associating liver partition and portal vein ligation for staged hepatectomy. J Gastrointest Surg 2017;21:967–974.
43 Serenari M, Collaud C, Alvarez FA, et al: Interstage assessment of remnant liver function in ALPPS using hepatobiliary scintigraphy. Ann Surg 2017;DOI: 10.1097/SLA.0000000000002150.
44 Pandanaboyana S, Bell R, Hidalgo E, et al: A systematic review and meta-analysis of portal vein ligation versus portal vein embolization for elective liver resection. Surgery 2015;157:690–698.
45 Li J, Kantas A, Ittrich H, et al: Avoid 'All-Touch' by hybrid ALPPS to achieve oncological efficacy. Ann Surg 2016;263:e6–7.
46 Donati M, Stavrou GA, Gulik TM, Oldhafer KJ: Associating liver partition and portal vein ligation for staged hepatectomy for Klatskin tumours: hinc sunt leones! ANZ J Surg 2015;85:3–4.
47 Adam R, Imai K, Castro Benitez C, et al: Outcome after associating liver partition and portal vein ligation for staged hepatectomy and conventional two-stage hepatectomy for colorectal liver metastases. Br J Surg 2016;103:1521–1529.
48 Dokmak S, Ftériche FS, Borscheid R, Cauchy F, Farges O, Belghiti J: 2012 Liver resections in the 21st century: we are far from zero mortality. HPB (Oxford) 2013;15:908–915.
49 Renfro LA, Goldberg RM, Grothey A, et al: Clinical calculator for early mortality in metastatic colorectal cancer: an analysis of patients from 28 clinical trials in the Aide et Recherche en Cancérologie Digestive Database. J Clin Oncol 2017;35:1929–1937.
50 Oldhafer KJ, Donati M, Jenner RM, Stang A, Stavrou GA: ALPPS for patients with colorectal liver metastases: effective liver hypertrophy, but early tumor recurrence. World J Surg 2014;38:1504–1509.
51 Schadde E, Ardiles V, Slankamenac K, et al: ALPPS offers a better chance of complete resection in patients with primarily unresectable liver tumors compared with conventional-staged hepatectomies: results of a multicenter analysis. World J Surg 2014;38:1510–1519.
52 Lang SA, Loss M, Benseler V, Glockzin G, Schlitt HJ: Long-term results after in-situ split (ISS) liver resection. Langenbecks Arch Surg 2015;400:361–369.
53 Lang H: ALPPS for colorectal liver metastases. J Gastrointest Surg 2017;21:190–192.
54 Björnsson B, Sparrelid E, Røsok B, et al: Associating liver partition and portal vein ligation for staged hepatectomy in patients with colorectal liver metastases – intermediate oncological results. Eur J Surg Oncol 2016;42:531–537.
55 Stintzing S, Miller-Phillips L, Modest DP, et al: Impact of BRAF and RAS mutations on first-line efficacy of FOLFIRI plus cetuximab versus FOLFIRI plus bevacizumab: analysis of the FIRE-3 (AIO KRK-0306) study. Eur J Cancer 2017;79:50–60.
56 Heinemann V, Weikersthal von LF, Decker T, et al: FOLFIRI plus cetuximab versus FOLFIRI plus bevacizumab as first-line treatment for patients with metastatic colorectal cancer (FIRE-3): a randomised, open-label, phase 3 trial. Lancet Oncol 2014;15:1065–1075.

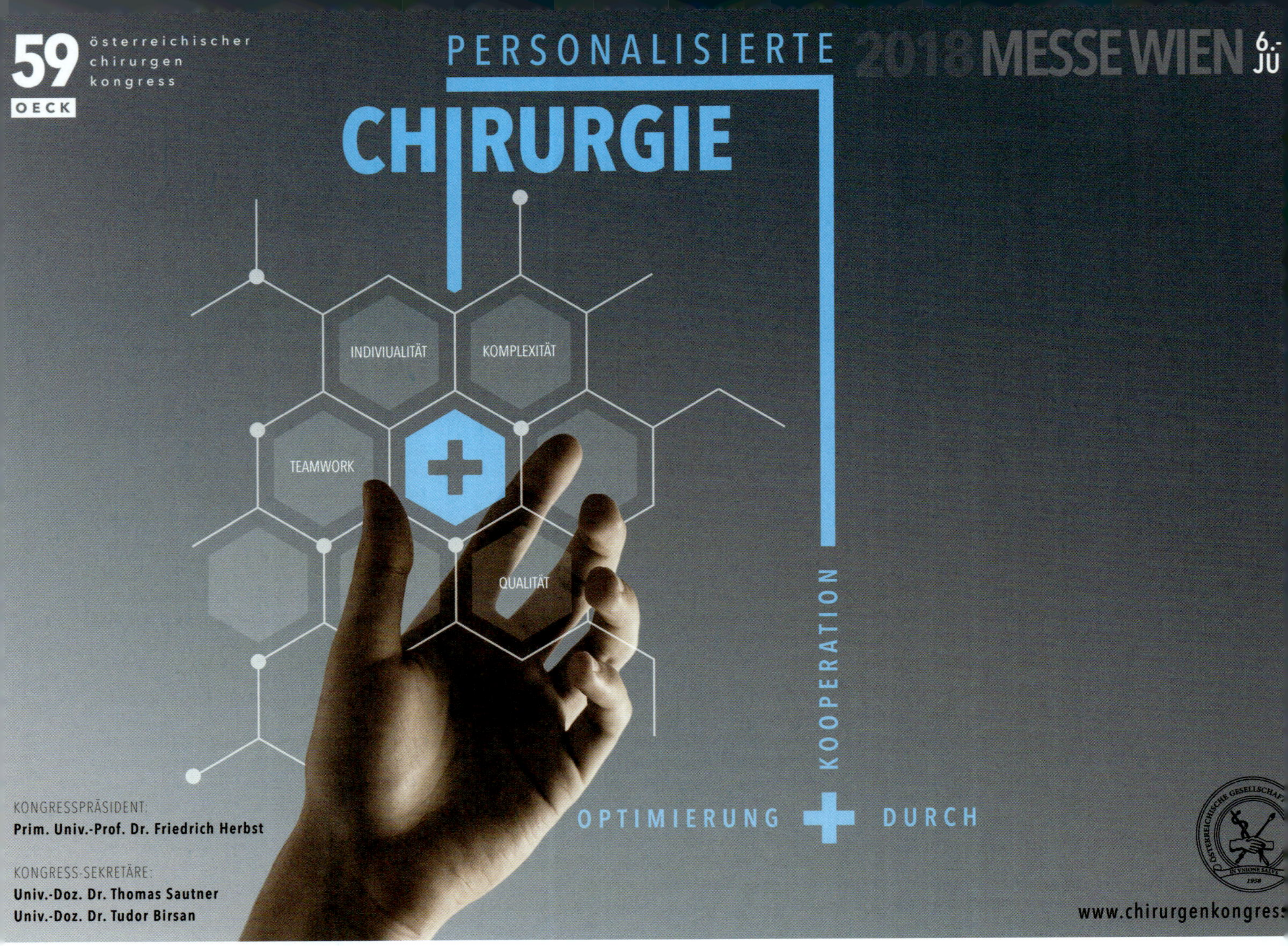
59
OECK
österreichischer
chirurgen
kongress
PERSONALISIERTE
CHIRURGIE
2018 MESSE WIEN
6.-
JU
INDIVIUALITÄT
KOMPLEXITÄT
TEAMWORK
QUALITÄT
KOOPERATION
OPTIMIERUNG
DURCH
KONGRESSPRÄSIDENT:
Prim. Univ.-Prof. Dr. Friedrich Herbst
KONGRESS-SEKRETÄRE:
Univ.-Doz. Dr. Thomas Sautner
Univ.-Doz. Dr. Tudor Birsan
www.chirurgenkongress

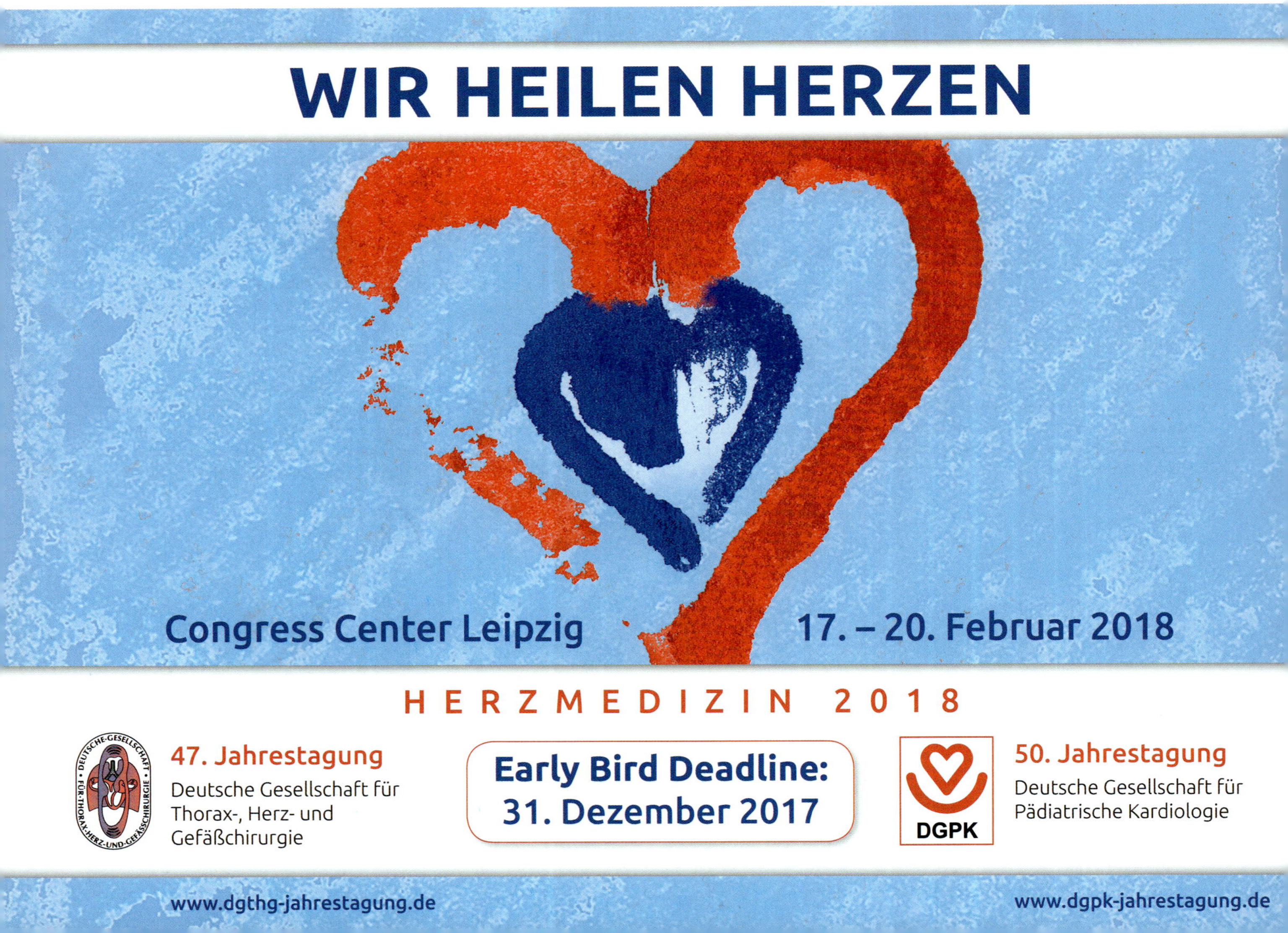
WIR HEILEN HERZEN
Congress Center Leipzig
17. – 20. Februar 2018
HERZMEDIZIN 2018
47. Jahrestagung
Deutsche Gesellschaft für
Thorax-, Herz- und
Gefäßchirurgie
Early Bird Deadline:
31. Dezember 2017
DGPK
50. Jahrestagung
Deutsche Gesellschaft für
Pädiatrische Kardiologie
www.dgthg-jahrestagung.de
www.dgpk-jahrestagung.de

Visceral Medicine

**Interdisciplinary Discussion**

Visc Med 2017;33:463–465
DOI: 10.1159/000485687

Published online: December 6, 2017

# Frontiers of Liver Surgery

Chair: Hauke Lang[a] Jens Mittler[a]

Participants: Karl J. Oldhafer[b,c] Erik Schadde[d–f] Yuzo Yamamoto[g]

[a] Department of General, Visceral, and Transplant Surgery, University Medical Center Mainz, Mainz, Germany;
[b] Department of General and Visceral Surgery, Surgical Oncology, Asklepios Klinik Barmbek, Hamburg, Germany;
[c] Semmelweis Medical Faculty, Campus Hamburg, Hamburg, Germany;
[d] Department of Surgery, Rush University Medical Center, Chicago, IL, USA;
[e] Cantonal Hospital Winterthur, Winterthur, Switzerland;
[f] Institute of Physiology, Center for Integrative Human Physiology, University of Zurich, Zurich, Switzerland;
[g] Department of Gastroenterological Surgery, Akita University Graduate School of Medicine, Akita, Japan

**Question 1: In patients requiring extended liver resection, when would you consider associating liver partition and portal vein ligation for staged hepatectomy (ALPPS) as opposed to preconditioning by portal vein embolization (PVE)? Does the underlying disease matter in your differential approach?**

*Oldhafer:* In my opinion, the first-line technique to obtain a sufficient future liver remnant (FLR) is PVE. It is very well established, and morbidity and mortality rates of the intervention are low. However, there are two important factors which need to be taken into consideration: First, a very low standardized FLR (sFLR), and second, a non- or low responder after PVE. In the first case, e.g. 15% FLR, I believe that a combination of PVE and ALPPS (so-called 'Hybrid-ALPPS') is a good tool to obtain a sufficient FLR. In my experience, the problem of a very low sFLR combined with a patient who underwent multiple cycles of chemotherapy will not be solved by PVE alone. In this case, dissection of the collaterals will greatly improve the regenerative capacity of the liver without increasing morbidity or mortality. Regarding the second factor, there are patients in daily clinical practice who will not respond adequately to PVE (also with segment 4 embolization). Therefore, the so-called 'Rescue-ALPPS' can achieve the desired volume.

As always, there are exceptions to the first statement in the first sentence. When considering ALPPS or PVE, metastases in the FLR will be an argument to perform a Hybrid-ALPPS. In this setting, we are able to free the FLR from tumor and transect the liver in one step and perform a PVE later.

Regarding the underlying cause, I refer to the second question and answer. However, the disease itself does not determine whether PVE or ALPPS is used.

*Schadde:* In my opinion, there is an absolute contraindication to use ALPPS in hepatocellular carcinoma (HCC) and cholangiocarcinoma, both intra- and extrahepatic, based on the evidence of catastrophic outcomes in the literature. From a medico-legal standpoint, its use for primary liver tumors cannot be justified at the moment. In contrast, it may be helpful in metastatic disease, in colorectal liver metastases (CRLM), in neuroendocrine tumors (NETs), and in NON-CR-NON-NET metastases.

The indications are extremely rare. 90% of patients can be appropriately treated with PVE or double embolization of the portal and hepatic veins. Its use may be justified for monosegment or double-segment FLR with a volume of less than 18%. In my opinion, its use is never justified to accelerate the resection, but only to increase the FLR volume. The second stage should not be done before 10 days have elapsed, and a HIDA scan to assess the function of the remnant liver is obligatory. I would not do a second stage with an Amsterdam index less than 3%/min/m$^2$. If you have a metastasis that is running away because it is not responding to chemotherapy or because it is growing too fast, then ALPPS will not save your patient. Surgery is not effective against tumor biology.

*Yamamoto:* I would select ALPPS when the cancer aggravation is impending. So far, I have tried ALPPS twice. The first case was in a patient with a giant HCC of 2,490 ml in the right liver. The volume of the liver remnant was only 350 ml (26.7%), and ICG-Krem was 0.037. The tumor was in a state of impending rupture, and the puncture route for percutaneous transhepatic PVE was difficult to obtain due to the huge tumor mass. One week post step 1 procedure, ICG-Krem had increased to 0.053. The second case was also in a patient with HCC of 774 ml in the right liver. The tumor was in a location broadly adhering to the inferior vena cava, and it

KARGER

Fax +49 761 4 52 07 14
Information@Karger.com
www.karger.com



Accessible online at:
www.karger.com/vis

Prof. Dr. med. Hauke Lang, MA, FACS
Klinik für Allgemein-, Viszeral- und Transplantationschirurgie
Universitätsmedizin Mainz
Langenbeckstraße 1, 55131 Mainz, Germany
Hauke.Lang@unimedizin-mainz.de

looked like the tumor was going to develop a tumor thrombus in the short hepatic veins soon.

I think that another indication for the ALPPS procedure is a patient in whom ICG-Krem is less than 0.04 because such patients often fail to increase ICG-Krem to over 0.05 even after PVE [1].

### Question 2: In your practice, where do you see contraindications to extended liver resection by ALPPS or resection following PVE? When do you choose not to operate on patients, namely those suffering from hilar cholangiocarcinoma?

*Oldhafer:* After the ALPPS meeting in 2015 in Hamburg, the data pointed clearly against liberal application of ALPPS in non-colorectal carcinoma (NCRC) patients. However, the first ALPPS itself was performed on a patient with an NCRC. Therefore, I think that ALPPS may play a role in patients with NCRC (e.g. hilar cholangiocarcinoma). Nevertheless, we need to think about the correct selection of patients.

Unfortunately, in daily practice, patients who suffer from hilar cholangiocarcinoma and who require extended right hepatectomies and PVE are often caught up in a diagnostic and interventional loop. Before thinking about hypertrophy concepts, they need to be drained (either by a percutaneous or endoscopic approach). The procedure itself can cause morbidity and mortality (cholangiosepsis, insufficient drainage). The time between drainage/PVE and resection can be very long and so much extended that at the time of the exploration, the tumor has already progressed.

This somehow answers the second part of the question: A patient with insufficient drainage, progress of the tumor, or low FLR will not be resected. Due to the insidious nature of hilar cholangiocarcinoma, however, surgical exploration will often be necessary to confirm the irresectability. In this setting, a palliative drainage operation can be considered.

*Schadde:* Absolute contraindications to ALPPS: all primary liver tumors, CRLM with progression on chemotherapy, breast, ovarian and testicular cancer metastases with progression on chemotherapy, neuroendocrine carcinoma (grade III NETs), NETs grade 1 and 2 with more than 10 lesions (complete resection too much, debulking suffices to prolong survival), fibrosis, cirrhosis, sinusoidal obstruction syndrome (SOS), chemotherapy-associated steatohepatitis (CASH), immune deficiency (e.g. s/p transplantation), history of more than 9 cycles of fluorouracil/platinum/irinotecan-based chemotherapies (those patients are eligible only to parenchymal-sparing resections).

Relative contraindications: age > 60 years (except for patients with a very good performance) as well as comorbidities that are prohibitive for major hepatectomies.

As far as hilar cholangiocarcinoma is concerned, extended resections are necessary in only a minority of patients in my opinion. Extended resections are only necessary in type IIIa/IIIb tumors with wide extension to the right and left side as well as type IV or intrahepatic cholangiocarcinomas in a hilar location, which in my opinion are not true Klatskin tumors. As long as the middle vein can be preserved (i.e., there is no tumor invasion into the middle hepatic vein), there is no reason to perform an extended resection.

ALPPS is contraindicated in cholangiocarcinoma; PVE always suffices to induce enough function in the FLR. I always perform a HIDA scan; bilirubin should be less than 1.5 mg/dl, otherwise resection is too risky.

*Yamamoto:* In my opinion, hilar cholangiocarcinoma is not a good indication for ALPPS because the manipulation of the hepatic hilum during the step 1 procedure hampers the non-touch isolation of the tumor. I choose PVE for hilar cholangiocarcinoma. If the patient does not gain an ICG-Krem > 0.05 by PVE, I will give up extended liver resection.

### Question 3: In your pre- and intraoperative decision making, when would you consider expanding your procedure by either vascular resection and reconstruction or multivisceral resection (e.g. hepatopancreatoduodenectomy) as opposed to aborting the procedure as an exploration?

*Oldhafer:* First, the physical performance and age of the patient play a pivotal role in extending the operation. However, an extended resection with vascular involvement will not be performed with certain tumor entities. Currently, in my opinion, if faced with a pancreatic carcinoma with vascular involvement, the patient needs to receive neoadjuvant therapy and to be included into a study, if eligible. If the extension of the vascular infiltration was underestimated preoperatively, the exploration needs to be terminated and we would refrain from resecting the tumor. Primary liver tumors, such as hilar cholangiocarcinomas, are usually associated with vascular infiltration; therefore, concomitant vascular resection can be anticipated. As stated before, the two most important aspects to extend the resection, either pre- or intraoperatively, are to consider the physical condition and performance of the patient and the tumor biology.

*Schadde:* Vascular resection: I have performed portal vein intra- and extrahepatic resections for hilar cholangiocarcinoma and metastatic disease. As a matter of principle I do not perform arterial resections and reconstructions in either hilar cholangiocarcinoma or CRLM, but I sometimes had to shave tumor off the artery. These are of course R1 resections except if there has been a complete response to chemotherapy. I have performed vena cava reconstructions with a 22 mm Gore-Tex ring graft, but these need to be planned ahead; that is never a matter of intraoperative decision making, especially when the hepatic veins are involved, due to veno-venous bypass and cooling. Imaging of the liver with magnetic resonance imaging as well as vascular and liver-specific contrast is so good that there is no need for intraoperative decision making here.

Extension into the duodenum is sometimes difficult to detect on imaging. I would never extend a major liver resection to a Whipple, but rather abort the procedure at the level of the exploration. The pancreatic head resection potentiates the risk of post-hepatectomy liver failure, and the liver resection potentiates the risk of Whipple complications. Both together are an explosive combination.

Part of the duodenum can on occasion be excised and closed when the liver tumor only invades the duodenum, but a Whipple is too much.

*Yamamoto:* When there is any possibility of R0 resection and tolerability of the patients, I usually try to expand the procedure. Vascular resection and reconstruction is usually not problematic, but I am cautious about hepatopancreatoduodenectomy due to possible serious complications.

## Question 4: Where do you see the future of laparoscopic and robotic liver surgery?

*Oldhafer:* I firmly believe that minimally invasive surgery in hepatobiliary surgery will be the future and needs to be trained and taught extensively. In diseases in which we are not sure whether the oncological outcome will reach that of the open procedure, the development of new technology and techniques will maybe even surpass the oncological open surgery in the years to come. However, in order to improve those two important factors, minimally invasive surgery needs to be implemented in high-volume centers. Then it will be possible to gather more prospective data and answer the questions regarding oncological equality.

*Schadde:* I think, if hepato-pancreato-biliary centers would stay up to date with existing skills and technology in 2017, 80% of all liver resections would be done laparoscopically in 2017, which is realistic, and that is what we currently do in Winterthur. That includes of course right and left hemi-hepatectomies, extended resections, resections after PVE and non-anatomic resections in segments 7, 8, 4a and 2 and biliary procedures like Roux-en-Y hepatico-jejunostomies. That should not be the future, but should be the present.

Big tumors, hilar tumors, and tumors requiring vascular reconstruction or bypass/cold perfusion will still be performed in an open fashion in 20 years from now.

The robotic technology will evolve. Eventually, everything that we are doing laparoscopically today will be done robotically in 20 years from now. Jumping from open to robotic without collecting experience with laparoscopy first is not a good idea in my opinion. Ultimately, however, I am sure that 90% of all surgery will be done robotically, like 90% of all airplanes are nowadays landed with the help of automatic landing systems.

*Yamamoto:* For complex liver resections, I do not see so much an advantage of laparoscopic surgery as the promoters say, but it will surely be incorporated as a trend of times. As to robotic surgery, apart from laparoscopic surgery, it might occupy an important position for reconstructing small vessels in liver surgery.

## References

1 Mihara T, Sugiura T, Okamura Y, et al: A predictive factor of insufficient liver regeneration after preoperative portal vein embolization. Eur Surg Res 2013;51:118–128.

## Participants

Prof. Dr. med. Karl J. Oldhafer
General and Visceral Surgery, Surgical Oncology
Asklepios Hospital Barmbek
Rübenkamp 220, 22291 Hamburg, Germany
k.oldhafer@asklepios.com

Erik Schadde, MD, FACS, FEBS (HPB)
Department of Surgery
Rush University Medical Center
1653 W. Congress Pkwy Jelke Building 7th Floor, 60612 Chicago, IL, USA
erik.schadde@uzh.ch

Yuzo Yamamoto, M.D., Ph.D.
Department of Gastroenterological Surgery
Akita University Graduate School of Medicine
1-1-1 Hondo, Akita 010-8543, Japan
yamamoto-kyt@umin.ac.jp

Visceral Medicine

**Clinical Therapeutic Review**

Visc Med 2017;33:466–476
DOI: 10.1159/000485014

Published online: December 8, 2017

# Intraductal Papillary Mucinous Neoplasms of the Pancreas: Strategic Considerations

Vicente Morales-Oyarvide  Zhi Ven Fong  Carlos Fernández-del Castillo  Andrew L. Warshaw

Department of Surgery, Massachusetts General Hospital and Harvard Medical School, Boston, MA, USA

**Keywords**
Intraductal papillary mucinous neoplasm, IPMN · Pancreatic cysts · Management

**Summary**
Intraductal papillary mucinous neoplasms (IPMN) are cystic neoplasms with the potential for progression to pancreatic cancer. Recognized by the global medical community just over two decades ago, IPMN have gained great epidemiological and clinical relevance thanks to the widespread use of cross-sectional abdominal imaging, which has led to a surge in the number of incidental pancreatic cysts being diagnosed. As our understanding of this disease has improved, we now know that some IPMN have a very elevated risk of cancer and require surgical resection, while others are low-risk lesions and can be followed. The approach to IPMN must therefore strike a balance between preventing the overutilization of surgery and the timely recognition and treatment of patients with high-risk lesions. Several clinical, radiographic, and laboratory parameters have been proposed to risk-stratify IPMN, leading to the publication of management guidelines that do not always converge in their recommendations. The goal of this clinical therapeutic review is to describe the strategic approach to IPMN at the Massachusetts General Hospital, and how our current understanding, management algorithm, and future directions have been informed by research efforts at our institution and other centers.



## Introduction

Intraductal papillary mucinous neoplasms (IPMN) have transformed the field of pancreatology. Regardless of the lens through which one approaches the study of the pancreas, the field as we know it today would be unrecognizable without IPMN and other pancreatic cystic neoplasms. Virtually unknown by the international medical community 25 years ago, IPMN account for nearly half of pancreatic resections for cystic lesions at the Massachusetts General Hospital (MGH) between 2005 and 2011 [1]. Our understanding of this disease has evolved dramatically over the past few decades. IPMN demonstrate a spectrum of cytomorphological atypia that is defined as low-grade dysplasia (LGD), high-grade dysplasia (HGD), and invasive carcinoma [2]. It is now clear that not all IPMN are the same: some affect the main pancreatic duct (MPD) extensively, have different clinical presentations, and pose a high risk of harboring an invasive carcinoma; while others remain confined to the side branches of the ductal system, are asymptomatic, and are considered low-risk lesions. Further, it is becoming ever more clear that invasive carcinomas arising from IPMN are distinct from 'conventional' pancreatic ductal adenocarcinomas (PDAC), demonstrating important morphological and genetic differences that have major prognostic implications [3–7].

The management of IPMN is complex; not too long ago, treatment approaches were based predominantly on institutional and individual experience. In 2004, a group of experts convened in Sendai, Japan, and drafted the first international consensus guidelines for the management of IPMN and mucinous cystic neoplasms (MCN) of the pancreas under the auspices of the International Association of Pancreatology (IAP) [8]. The IAP Sendai consensus guidelines (as they became known) were the first international effort to standardize treatment and follow-up for patients with this condition. A few years later and after several validation studies, these guidelines were updated following a meeting in Fukuoka, Japan, and the IAP 2012 Fukuoka consensus guidelines became the

KARGER

Fax +49 761 4 52 07 14
Information@Karger.com
www.karger.com



Accessible online at:
www.karger.com/vis

Andrew L. Warshaw, M.D.
Department of Surgery
Massachusetts General Hospital
55 Fruit St., BUL370, Boston, MA 02114, USA
awarshaw@partners.org

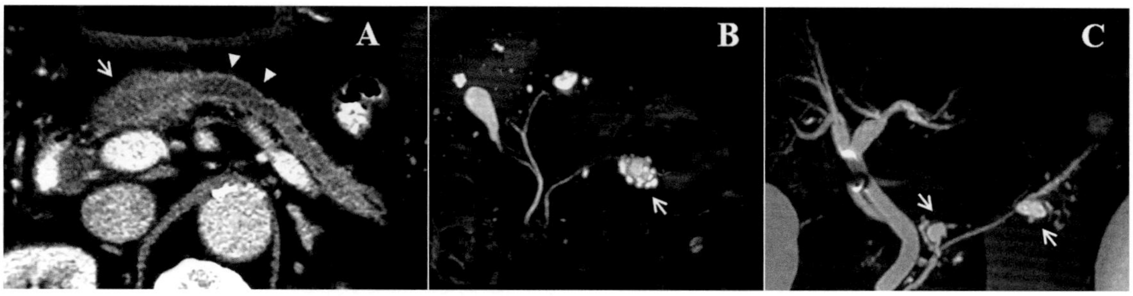


**Fig. 1.** Intraductal papillary mucinous neoplasm (IPMN) types based on main pancreatic duct (MPD) involvement. **A** Main duct IPMN; contrast-enhanced computed tomography showing a heterogeneous, hypodense lesion in the pancreatic neck (arrow) with dilation of the MPD (arrow heads) and distal atrophy. **B** Branch duct IPMN; magnetic resonance with cholangiopancreatography (MRCP) demonstrating a T2 hyperintense lesion (arrow) in the pancreatic body showing communication with the MPD. **C** Mixed-type IPMN; MRCP revealing cystic lesions in the head and body of the pancreas, communicating with the MPD (arrows); involvement of the MPD is not apparent on radiographic imaging but was found on histological examination after resection (mixed-type IPMN with minimal histological involvement of the MPD).

preponderant set of recommendations [9]. The safety and efficacy of these guidelines has been assessed extensively, and they were further revised in 2017, with only minor modifications [10].

With increased awareness and widespread use of cross-sectional abdominal imaging, the number of patients diagnosed with pancreatic cysts has only continued to grow and it has become a preeminent issue for the gastroenterological community. As a result, in 2015, the American Gastroenterological Association (AGA) put forth the AGA Institute guidelines on the diagnosis and management of pancreatic cysts [11] following an exhaustive technical review of the literature [12]. As we will discuss later in this article, the IAP and AGA guidelines exhibit critical contrasts that reflect our still limited understanding of the natural history of IPMN and how much more we must learn. At MGH, we have strived to be at the cutting edge of the research efforts to better understand the biology and behavior of IPMN, and while we have mostly followed the IAP guidelines in our clinical practice, our perspective may not always align with every aspect of the latest international consensus. Our goal in this article is to provide an overview of the MGH institutional experience with IPMN and of how our research – often in collaboration with other centers – has helped to inform our strategic approach to these tumors.

## Epidemiology of Intraductal Papillary Mucinous Neoplasms

The true prevalence of IPMN is not known, but the generalized use of cross-sectional imaging has allowed us to conclude that pancreatic cysts become common with increasing age [13, 14]. Calculating the prevalence of incidental (i.e. asymptomatic) pancreatic cysts in the general population is a complex task, as most studies have included patients from tertiary care centers who may have a history of liver or pancreatobiliary conditions, thus introducing potential for referral bias [14, 15]. To overcome this limitation, a study by de Jong et al. [16] assessed the prevalence of pancreatic cysts in 2,803 consecutive subjects (mean age 51.1 years) who underwent screening with abdominal magnetic resonance imaging (MRI) as part of a preventive medical examination. The authors identified pancreatic cysts in 2.4% of the subjects, and their presence was strongly correlated with age: less than 1% of subjects between 18 and 49 years of age had a pancreatic cyst, compared to 10% of individuals older than 70 years. Importantly, most cysts were smaller than 1 cm (median size 8 mm), with only a few being larger than 2 cm; among patients with pancreatic cysts, 12% were multifocal. There is no robust evidence on the exact pathological diagnosis of these asymptomatic pancreatic cysts, but it is believed that a large proportion of them are small IPMN confined to the ductal side branches. While IPMN have traditionally been considered more common in men, especially in surgical series, there was no gender difference in the observed prevalence of pancreatic cysts. Our institutional experience is consistent with the above findings in relation to patient age and sex: the median age at initial diagnosis of 577 patients with suspected or presumed IPMN undergoing surveillance at MGH was 66 years, and 59% were women [17].

## Types of Intraductal Papillary Mucinous Neoplasms Based on Main Pancreatic Duct Involvement: The First Layer of Classification

IPMN are primarily classified as main duct (MD-IPMN), branch duct (BD-IPMN), or mixed-type IPMN based on the extent to which they involve the pancreatic ductal system (fig. 1). Preoperatively, this distinction is defined by the diameter of the MPD on imaging studies: according to the revised IAP 2012 Fukuoka consensus guidelines [10], segmental or diffuse dilation of the MPD of >5 mm without other causes of obstruction defines MD-IPMN (fig. 1A); pancreatic cysts >5 mm in size demonstrating communication with the MPD but with no MPD dilation are classified as BD-IPMN (fig. 1B); and lesions meeting criteria for both MD- and BD-IPMN are classified as mixed-type IPMN. This classification is of biological and practical importance: based on a summary of 20 different studies including 3,568 IPMN, the risk of invasive carcinoma arising in association with MD-IPMN is approximately 44%, compared to approximately 17% in BD-IPMN [9]. These estimates vary widely across centers, in part because some studies classify tumors based on their degree of histological – rather than radiological – MPD involvement, and the two criteria have shown a modest correlation (approximately 70%) [18, 19]. In our institution, the

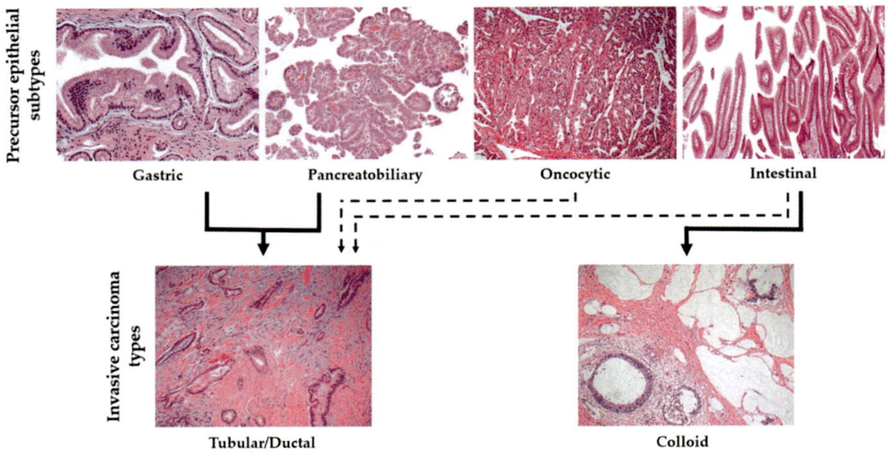


**Fig. 2.** The precursor and invasive components of intraductal papillary mucinous neoplasms (IPMN) demonstrate morphological and genetic heterogeneity. Based on its cytoarchitectural features, the precursor component is classified as gastric, pancreatobiliary, oncocytic, or intestinal. Invasive carcinomas arising from gastric- and pancreatobiliary-type IPMN exhibit a tubular/ductal morphology, similar to that of conventional pancreatic ductal adenocarcinoma; in comparison, most invasive carcinomas arising from intestinal-type IPMN are of the colloid type. Oncocytic-type IPMN can give rise to invasive carcinoma, either superficially invasive, of tubular type, or of oncocytic type.

risk of HGD and invasive carcinoma in resected, radiologically defined MD-IPMN is 32 and 47%, respectively; in comparison, the risk of HGD and invasive carcinoma in resected BD-IPMN is 15 and 9%. We must emphasize that these risk estimates derive from resected IPMN; since most BD-IPMN are not resected, their actual risk of HGD and invasive carcinoma must be much lower. Naturally, these differences in risk between MD- and BD-IPMN have a huge influence on the treatment strategy for each IPMN type: based on the revised IAP 2012 Fukuoka consensus guidelines [10], radiological MPD involvement is an indication for resection in surgically fit patients; in comparison, patients with BD-IPMN may be offered surgery or surveillance based on the presence of clinical and radiological worrisome features and high-risk stigmata, as we will detail later in this article.

Mixed-type IPMN, on the other hand, have been a source of growing interest in recent years. They have historically been considered akin to MD-IPMN (the revised 2012 Fukuoka consensus guidelines recommend identical management for both types), but evidence suggests that not all mixed-type IPMN are equal. At MGH, mixed-type IPMN defined by current imaging criteria have a risk of HGD and invasive carcinoma of 31 and 28%, respectively: higher than that of BD-IPMN, but lower than MD-IPMN. Detailed histological analysis of these tumors by our group has shed light on this 'mixed' behavior [20]. Pathological re-review of 404 resected IPMN revealed that some mixed-type IPMN (approximately 1 of every 5) demonstrate only minimal histological involvement of the MPD (non-circumferential microscopic involvement), and this subgroup had a risk of HGD (11%) and invasive carcinoma (6%) comparable to that of histologically-defined BD-IPMN (fig. 1C); in contrast, mixed-type IPMN with extensive MPD involvement had a significantly higher risk of HGD (37%) and invasive carcinoma (33%). These data suggest that mixed-type IPMN with minimal histological MPD involvement may have a more indolent behavior and could perhaps be managed in a similar way as BD-IPMN. At this point, the distinction between mixed-type IPMN with minimal versus extensive histological MPD involvement can only be made after surgery, when it is only of little relevance compared with the identification of invasive carcinoma, but preliminary data from our institution indicate that preoperative recognition of histological MPD involvement may be feasible. We found that MPD diameter as measured by computed tomography (CT) or MRI is effective at distinguishing extensive versus minimal histological MPD involvement (area under the curve (AUC) 0.85; 95% confidence interval (CI) 0.80–0.90) [21].

## Epithelial Subtypes of the Precursor Component and the Invasive Carcinoma: Insights into Tumor Biology and Its Heterogeneity

IPMN are characterized by papillary formations that project into the pancreatic ductal system. The epithelial lining of these papillae displays significant morphologic heterogeneity that has led to the recognition of four distinct epithelial subtypes of the precursor component (i.e. non-invasive component), namely: gastric, intestinal, pancreatobiliary, and oncocytic (fig. 2) [22, 23]. Since it is not rare to encounter more than one epithelial subtype in each tumor, IPMN are classified based on the predominant subtype. Invasive carcinomas arising from IPMN also exhibit important histological differences and are classified as tubular (ductal), colloid, and oncocytic types (fig. 2) [22, 23]. The recognition of different precursor and invasive phenotypes has important prognostic implications, and it is becoming increasingly clear that these subgroups may represent specific pathways of differentiation with distinct molecular features [5, 6, 24]. Gastric-type epithelium is most common in BD-IPMN and is often associated with LGD (77% of resected gastric-type IPMN at our institution); paradoxically, when invasive carcinoma arises from a gastric-type IPMN, it is usually of tubular type, which carries a poor prognosis akin to that of conventional PDAC [3]. As in PDAC, *KRAS* mutations are highly prevalent in gastric-type IPMN and tubular-type carcinomas [25, 26]. In contrast, intestinal-type epithelium is predominantly found in MD-IPMN, is associated with HGD and invasive carcinoma (40 and 33% of intestinal-type IPMN at our institution, respectively), and often gives rise to colloid-type carcinoma, which has more favorable clinicopathological features and prognosis [3]. Moreover, intestinal-type IPMN and colloid-type carcinomas exhibit *GNAS* mutations and markers of intestinal differentiation (e.g. MUC2 positivity and *CDX2* expression) [24–26]. Pancreatobiliary-type epithelium is uncommon (<5% of IPMN resections at MGH), and in many cases it is hard to distinguish from gastric-type IPMN with HGD [23]; it virtually always demonstrates HGD or invasive carcinoma (47 and 53% at our institution, respectively), and when it is invasive it gives rise to tubular-type carcinomas. Of the four epithelial subtypes, oncocytic-type IPMN is perhaps the most unique. Highly infrequent (accounting for only 4% of resections at MGH), this subtype is associated with MPD involvement, HGD, and invasive carcinoma of the oncocytic type, but has surprisingly favorable outcomes: in a series of 18 patients from our hospital, the median overall survival (OS) after resection was more than 10 years and there were no disease-specific deaths [27]. Given the above considerations, the revised IAP 2012 Fukuoka consensus guidelines emphasize the importance of classifying invasive carcinomas arising from IPMN as tubular, colloid, or oncocytic [10], and this is our standard practice. Whether the different types of invasive carcinoma exhibit distinct response to adjuvant chemotherapy and radiation remains unclear, and we need more research on this topic to continue tailoring patient treatment and follow-up.

We recently reported that age plays a role in IPMN heterogeneity [28]. In a series of 1,693 resected IPMN from the institutions conforming the Pancreatic Surgery Consortium (MGH, Memorial Sloan Kettering Cancer Center, and the Johns Hopkins Hospital), we found that IPMN from patients who were younger than 50 years of age at the time of resection were more likely to be of the oncocytic and intestinal subtypes; moreover, they were less likely to harbor an invasive carcinoma, and when this was present, it was more often of colloid type and associated with improved OS. We continued to observe these associations – albeit in lesser magnitude – using age cutoffs of 55 and 60 years of age. Notably, only 5% of patients undergoing resection were younger than 50, a fact that underscores the tremendous importance of multi-center collaborations if we are to characterize uncommon subsets of patients that would otherwise be too rare in single-center series.

## Clinical Presentation

We will next discuss the different information and tools available for identifying patients with high-risk lesions. Most IPMN currently being diagnosed are asymptomatic (i.e. incidental), especially BD-IPMN. In a series of 563 BD-IPMN (411 primarily observed and 152 primarily resected) from our institution, 57% were asymptomatic [29]. In a follow-up study limited to patients with a minimum of 6 months of surveillance (i.e. excluding those who were offered surgery soon after diagnosis), 83% were asymptomatic at initial diagnosis, and of these, only 10% went on to become symptomatic during follow-up [17]. As one would expect, the rate of symptomatic IPMN is higher in surgical series. Half of patients who have undergone resection for IPMN at MGH were symptomatic, with the most common symptom being abdominal pain (41%), followed by weight loss >10 lbs (29%), acute pancreatitis (22%), and jaundice (9%).

Diabetes mellitus – especially of recent onset – is a common finding in patients with conventional PDAC [30], but its role as a harbinger of HGD and invasive carcinoma in IPMN has not been well studied. We recently reported that diabetes mellitus is common among patients undergoing resection for IPMN (34%), and it is associated with a twofold elevated risk of HGD and invasive carcinoma (analyzed as separate endpoints) after adjusting for IAP 2012 Fukuoka worrisome features [31]. Moreover, recent-onset diabetes mellitus (diagnosed ≤5 years before surgery) was associated with 6.9-fold increased risk of invasive carcinoma ($p < 0.001$). If further studies validate the independent role of diabetes mellitus in the prediction of HGD and invasive carcinoma in IPMN, it could be considered an additional element of the management algorithm.

In addition to being associated with degree of dysplasia, some symptoms of presentation may be informative of the IPMN epithelial subtypes. We have reported that IPMN from patients presenting with acute pancreatitis are 4.8 times more likely to be of the intestinal subtype [32]. Similarly, a diagnosis of diabetes mellitus is associated with 1.6-fold and 2.5-fold higher likelihood of intestinal-type IPMN and colloid-type carcinoma, respectively [31]. As we discussed previously, intestinal-type IPMN usually involve the MPD and secrete MUC2-rich, viscous mucin. We hypothesize that these thick secretions may lead to duct obstruction and pancreatic inflammation, which could be associated with episodes of acute pancreatitis and perhaps with development of diabetes mellitus, but at this point this is merely speculative.

## Circulating Biomarkers for Prediction of High-Risk Intraductal Papillary Mucinous Neoplasms

Multiple circulating biomarkers have been assessed as potential indicators of HGD or invasive carcinoma in IPMN. Of those, the most widely studied is the carbohydrate antigen 19-9 (CA 19-9), an independent predictor of disease stage and survival in patients with resectable, conventional PDAC [33]. In a recent meta-analysis of fifteen studies and a total of 1,629 patients [34], elevated serum CA 19-9 had a pooled sensitivity and specificity of 52 and 88% for detecting invasive carcinoma in IPMN, respectively. Unfortunately, the authors did not conduct analyses using HGD without invasive carcinoma as a separate study endpoint. Data from our institution [35] indicate that serum CA 19-9 in patients with resected BD-IPMN is useful for detecting invasive carcinoma (AUC 0.68; 95% CI 0.52–0.84) but not for detecting HGD without invasive carcinoma (AUC 0.54; 95% CI 0.42–0.67). Importantly, a cutoff of 100 units/ml had the highest accuracy for detecting invasive carcinoma (93%), compared with the more commonly used cutoff of 37 units/ml (83%) [36, 37]. Elevated serum CA 19-9 has now been included as a worrisome feature in the revised IAP 2012 Fukuoka consensus guidelines [10]; while our experience would support this addition, we must keep in mind that its utility appears to be restricted to detecting invasive carcinoma (and not HGD), and the optimal cutoff value may still need to be determined.

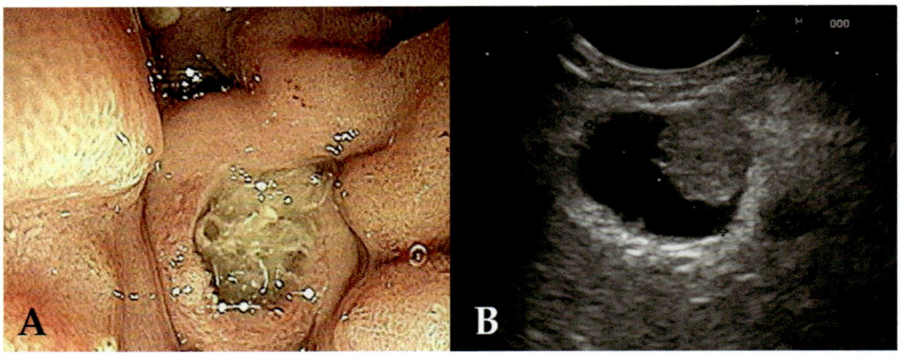

**Fig. 3.** Endoscopic and ultrasonographic evaluation of intraductal papillary mucinous neoplasms (IPMN). **A** Upper endoscopy demonstrating a patulous, 'fish-mouth' papilla extruding mucus, pathognomonic of IPMN affecting the main pancreatic duct. **B** Endoscopic ultrasound revealing a mural nodule within the cyst, a known harbinger of high-grade dysplasia and invasive carcinoma in IPMN.

More recently, the neutrophil-to-lymphocyte ratio (NLR) in blood has been evaluated as a novel predictor of HGD and invasive carcinoma, which could presumably reflect the systemic immune response elicited by cancer, among other potential physiologic mechanisms [38, 39]. In a series of 272 patients with resected IPMN from the Johns Hopkins Hospital, Gemenetzis et al. [39] found that an NLR > 4 was significantly associated with invasive carcinoma, independent of MPD size, presence of mural nodules, jaundice, and cyst size. Notably, a higher NLR was not associated with HGD without invasive carcinoma. At our institution, we do not systematically use blood NLR in the assessment of patients with IPMN, but we recognize its practical potential as a biomarker and the need for validation studies. Similar to serum CA 19-9, its main shortcoming lies in the limited ability to detect HGD without invasive carcinoma.

## Imaging Evaluation

Different cross-sectional and ultrasonographic imaging modalities are used in the initial assessment and surveillance of patients with IPMN, each with its own strengths and limitations. Imaging studies pursue two primary goals: to distinguish IPMN from other pancreatic cysts, and to identify MPD involvement to determine IPMN with higher risk of harboring HGD or invasive carcinoma. Multidetector CT (MDCT) and MRI with cholangiopancreatography (MRCP) are effective and reliable methods to characterize cyst morphology, size, and communication with the MPD. In our experience, MDCT and MRCP can distinguish mucinous versus non-mucinous cysts with an accuracy of 71–85% [40, 41]. The risk assessment of lesions suspected to be IPMN is centered on the recognition of MPD involvement and presence of mural nodules within or adjacent to the cyst, both known markers of HGD and invasive carcinoma. Accurately identifying mural nodules has proven to be a challenge, since they are often hard to distinguish from mucin plugs. In an effort to further understand the evaluation of mural nodules, studies have shown that nodule size can help identify patients at higher risk of HGD and invasive carcinoma [42, 43]. In the original IAP 2012 Fukuoka consensus guidelines, presence of an enhancing mural nodule was defined as a high-risk stigma without further consideration of nodule size; the new revised IAP 2012 Fukuoka consensus guidelines recommend that mural nodules ≥5 mm be considered a high-risk stigma, while a size smaller than 5 mm be regarded as a worrisome feature [10]. More research is needed to determine whether we should be concerned about the size of mural nodules, and if so, what the optimal size threshold is.

Our experience and that of other centers show that both MDCT (especially dual-phase pancreatic protocol CT) and gadolinium-enhanced MRI are adequate for initial evaluation and surveillance of suspected IPMN, with an accuracy to identify lesions with HGD and invasive carcinoma in the range of 75–86% in two contemporary studies from our institution [40, 41, 44]. While both imaging modalities have demonstrated comparable diagnostic performance [40, 44], MRI is favored as the method of choice for surveillance of suspected IPMN [45]. This is partly because MRI may allow for superior visualization of the ductal system anatomy, presence of internal septations, and mural nodules, but more importantly because it spares patients under long-term surveillance from repeated radiation exposure that would otherwise occur with MDCT.

Various endoscopic modalities are used to further characterize suspected IPMN. Upper endoscopy can reveal the classic, patulous 'fish mouth' papilla extruding mucus, which is pathognomonic of IPMN involving the MPD (fig. 3A) [46, 47], although the trend towards early diagnosis of small, incidental lesions has made this finding increasingly rare. Endoscopic retrograde cholangiopancreatography with or without pancreatoscopy has been used to obtain pancreatic juice and brushings for cytology, and to visualize papillary or villous growths along the ducts, but evidence to support its routine use is lacking and we do not recommend it [10, 47]. Endoscopic ultrasound (EUS) has become a highly valuable tool in the diagnostic work-up of IPMN; guidelines make different recommendations regarding who should be investigated with this technique, as we will discuss in a later section. One of the advantages of EUS is its superior ability to detect mural nodules, one of the stronger predictors of high-risk IPMN (fig. 3B), albeit with risk of false positives due to the mucin plugs mentioned earlier [48–50]. This caveat can be avoided using contrast-enhanced harmonic EUS, which allows the operator to reliably detect blood flow in the suspected nodule and thus to better distinguish mucin plugs from true mural nodules with a sensitivity and specificity of 89–96% and 64–88%, respectively [51]. Beyond the detailed characterization of IPMN morphology, EUS offers another diagnostic advantage: it allows us to perform EUS-guided fine-needle aspiration of the cyst contents, paving the way for comprehensive cyst fluid analysis and cytology.

## Cyst Fluid Analysis: Proteins, Cytology, and Molecular Characterization

Our understanding of pancreatic cyst fluid analysis continues to evolve and, for the most part, remains investigational. For the purposes of this discussion, we will classify the different cyst fluid parameters of interest as cyst fluid protein (antigen) analysis, cytological analysis, and molecular analysis. Carcinoembryonic antigen (CEA) is the most widely studied protein marker in pancreatic cyst fluid. It cannot distinguish between benign cysts and those with HGD or invasive carcinoma [52], but it is very valuable to distinguish mucinous from non-mucinous lesions. A cooperative study between MGH and several other centers found in 2004 that a CEA cutoff value of 192 ng/ml had the greatest AUC (0.79; accuracy 79%) to detect mucinous cysts [53]. A more recent study including nearly twice as many patients from our institution showed that a cutoff value of 109.9 ng/ml is more accurate (86%) and has a greater AUC (0.93) [54]. Neither the IAP nor the AGA guidelines set cyst fluid CEA thresholds in their recommendations, but 192 ng/ml remains the most consistently used value.

In a collaborative effort with the Rutgers Robert Wood Johnson Medical School, we have also found that mAb Das-1, a monoclonal antibody that reacts specifically with normal colonic epithelium and intestinal metaplasia of the lower esophagus (Barrett's esophagus), can identify high-risk IPMN using cyst fluid with a sensitivity and specificity of 89 and 100%, respectively [55]. A preliminary, multi-institutional validation study of the performance of mAb Das-1 confirmed our initial findings and suggests that this antibody may be a valuable addition to current clinical guidelines [56].

The interpretation of cyst fluid cytological and molecular analyses presents a greater challenge. Even in referral centers with highly specialized endoscopists and cytopathologists, the sensitivity of pancreatic cyst fluid cytology is low due to insufficient aspirated volume, scant cellularity, and contamination with gastric and duodenal mucosal cells. These hurdles make it difficult to reach a formal determination of 'positive' cytology. Cytopathologists from our institution have shown that lowering the threshold from 'positive' cytology to presence of high-grade atypical epithelial cells (which are quantitatively and qualitatively insufficient for a positive cytology interpretation), we can achieve an increase in the accuracy (80–85%) and in the number of cases of HGD and invasive carcinoma detected (12% more than when using 'positive' cytology) [57, 58]. Lastly, the continuous progress in genomic technologies holds the promise of accurate diagnosis and risk stratification of pancreatic cysts using molecular analysis of cyst fluid. Most studies have focused on determining alterations in *KRAS* and *GNAS,* two of the more common gene alterations in IPMN; the former are considered highly specific of mucinous lesions (also occurring in some MCN) and are found in the fluid of approximately half of IPMN, while the latter are believed to be specific of IPMN (especially so in those demonstrating intestinal-colloid differentiation) and are observed in the cyst fluid of approximately two thirds of IPMN (mutations in either gene are detected in 45–96% of IPMN) [5, 26, 59]. Unfortunately, regardless of how sensitive or specific mutations in these genes may be for differentiating IPMN from other cystic lesions, they do not inform risk of HGD or invasive carcinoma. Recent efforts from our center and others have shown that performing next-generation sequencing in fluid from pancreatic cysts is feasible [60], allowing for the identification of mutations in several genes whose exact role in diagnosis and management is still undetermined but may prove very useful in the near future.

Ultimately, the information we obtain from protein, cytological, and molecular analyses of cyst fluid will be part of a larger mosaic that incorporates a patient's clinical picture, serum markers, and imaging findings. Indeed, a recent multi-center study from several countries offered promising results using a combination of clinical features and molecular markers, allowing for determination of pancreatic cyst type with a sensitivity of 90–100% and specificity of 92–98% [61].

## Considerations Regarding Operative Approach to Intraductal Papillary Mucinous Neoplasms

Patients with completely resected non-invasive (i.e. LGD or HGD) IPMN have excellent outcomes, with >95% 10-year disease-specific survival [62]. In contrast, patients with resected invasive carcinoma have a poor prognosis, with 5- and 10-year OS rates of 47 and 34%, respectively, in our experience [3]. Among these, outcomes differ based on the type of invasive carcinoma: tubular-type carcinoma is associated with 5-year OS rates of 37%, whereas 5-year OS for colloid carcinoma is approximately 61% [3]. These survival estimates clearly demonstrate that IPMN need to be diagnosed and resected at an early stage; they also show that the distinction between HGD and invasive carcinoma is of paramount importance. This distinction is not clear in many studies, limiting our ability to compare different series and putting two groups of patients with wide contrasts in one basket. While we are not certain about the natural history of IPMN with HGD, waiting for invasive carcinoma to develop in a disease as lethal as pancreatic cancer would render our surveillance efforts pointless. We therefore strongly recommend that studies evaluating potential new markers for risk stratification of IPMN analyze HGD and invasive carcinoma as two separate endpoints, with a strong emphasis on HGD.

Mortality associated with pancreatic resection has decreased substantially. In the last two decades, surgical-related death after a pancreatoduodenectomy at MGH occurred in 1.5% of patients, with septic shock being the most common cause of death (33%) [63]. Surgical morbidity, however, remains an issue. Up to 45% of patients undergoing surgery for IPMN suffer from a complication (e.g. delayed gastric emptying, wound infection, cardiopulmonary complications), with 12% of complications being pancreatic fistulas. Despite the high morbidity rate, patients undergoing pancreatoduodenectomy eventually report high health-related quality of life and functional status 5 years after the procedure [64].

The presence of comorbidities is an important consideration when deciding in which patients to recommend pancreatic resection. Patients with a high comorbidity burden who are at high risk of non-IPMN-related death may derive little to no benefit from active surveillance or pancreatic surgery. Using the age-adjusted Charlson comorbidity index (CACI), we found that in a group of 725 patients who underwent resection or were under surveillance for IPMN at MGH, the median CACI score was 3 [65]. 10% of patients had a CACI ≥ 7 (indicating severe comorbidities), and their median OS was 43 months. Compared to patients with a CACI < 7, those with a CACI ≥ 7 had an 11-fold higher risk of dying from non-IPMN-related causes within 3 years. Thus, patients with severe comorbidity burden are at greater risk of non-IPMN-related death, even in the presence of invasive carcinoma. Based on these findings, neither active surveillance nor resection would be justified in this subgroup.

The standard surgical approach for patients with IPMN meeting indications for resection is pancreatoduodenectomy, left (distal) pancreatectomy, or total pancreatectomy depending on the location and extension of the tumor, all accompanied by lymph node dissection [10]. A growing number of studies has recently advocated for increased consideration of limited, non-anatomic resections (e.g. enucleation, middle pancreatectomy) for some instances of BD-IPMN. These parenchymal-sparing approaches may manage to preserve pancreatic exocrine and endocrine function, albeit sometimes with high rates of short-term surgical morbidity [66–68]. From our perspective, the idea of performing enucleation of a tumor communicating with the MPD is problematic (i.e., by definition, all IPMN). If it is felt that an IPMN poses an elevated risk of HGD or invasive carcinoma and needs to be resected, then enucleation would not be a sound approach from an oncologic standpoint. Additionally, if the risk of HGD or invasive carcinoma is thought to be so low that enucleation would be an appropriate procedure, that patient should not have undergone any pancreatic resection in the first place. Considerations about the 'radicality' of surgery (i.e. resection margin status, IPMN left behind in the remnant pancreas) will be discussed in the next section in the context of follow-up after resection and prediction of disease recurrence.

## Follow-up of Resected Patients: Predicting Recurrent and New Lesions

Disease recurrence remains a concern after primary resection for IPMN. We define recurrence as presence of new IPMN on imaging studies, either i) at the resection margin of the primary surgery or ii) in the pancreas remnant, peripancreatic lymph nodes, or distant organs. Known ('residual') IPMN located away from the resection margin and purposefully left behind during primary surgery are not recurrent lesions and should be assessed individually. As in most other matters involved in the management and outcomes of patients with IPMN, the risk of recurrence depends heavily on the degree of MPD involvement and on the presence of invasive carcinoma in the resected tumor. In our experience, the overall recurrence rate for resected IPMN is around 17%, and of those patients, around 14% require a second surgery [69]. The relatively low rate of reoperation in patients who recur is because not all recurrences are equal: some IPMN recur in the form of an invasive carcinoma, while others do so as non-invasive lesions. Nearly half of patients undergoing resection for IPMN with invasive carcinoma experience recurrence within a median of 19 months, which is virtually always invasive. These recurrences occur more commonly in patients with lymph node metastases and in those with tubular-type carcinomas. Conversely, less than 10% of non-invasive IPMN recur, and in the case of non-invasive BD-IPMN, the recurrence is almost always a non-invasive lesion and occurs after a median of more than 4 years after primary resection. Consequently, and in accordance with the revised IAP 2012 Fukuoka consensus guidelines, we recommend that patients undergoing resection for IPMN with invasive carcinoma should continue surveillance similar to that of conventional PDAC [10].

The follow-up of patients with resected, non-invasive IPMN is more controversial. Our experience shows that approximately 9% of non-invasive IPMN recur, consistent with other referral centers that have reported recurrence rates of 5–8% in this patient subgroup [70, 71]. Furthermore, it is becoming clearer that IPMN are associated with a 'field defect', whereby the entire pancreas would be affected and at higher risk of pancreatic neoplasia, a hypothesis driven in part by the occurrence of synchronous, multifocal disease and concomitant (concurrent) PDAC arising separately from IPMN. In our experience, up to 47% of BD-IPMN are multifocal and the number of lesions was more than four in as many as 18% of patients [29]. There is no conclusive evidence that multifocal IPMN pose a higher risk of HGD or invasive carcinoma, and we thus recommend that each cyst be assessed individually, rather than performing a total pancreatectomy upfront [10, 48, 72]. More critically, concomitant PDAC may develop in 3–11% of patients, either in the primary resection specimen or as a metachronous event [73–75]. While our experience suggests that metachronous PDAC after resection for IPMN is uncommon (0.5%), other series have reported a 5- and 10-year cumulative incidence of 4.5 and 5.9%, respectively [76]. Hence, we also support continuing surveillance of surgically fit patients after resection of non-invasive IPMN [10].

The importance of achieving a clear resection margin to prevent disease recurrence is controversial. It is widely accepted that clear evidence of HGD or invasive carcinoma at the resection margin is a very strong predictor of disease recurrence and warrants further surgical resection [10, 69]. The clinical relevance of LGD at the resection margins, however, is not well established. In our institutional experience, approximately 16% of patients had positive resection margins (71% in the form of LGD, 15% HGD, and 14% invasive carcinoma), and this group had a significantly higher risk of recurrence compared with patients with negative margins (25 vs. 14%, $p = 0.008$) [69]. Our findings are largely consistent with a study from Memorial Sloan Kettering Cancer Center [77], in which the presence of IPMN (LGD or HGD) or pancreatic intraepithelial neoplasia at the resection margins was significantly associated with disease recurrence; nevertheless, the vast majority of recurrences did not occur at the resection margins but elsewhere in the pancreatic remnant. Thus, if the rationale for extended resections with margins clear of LGD is to prevent recurrent disease at the resection margin, current evidence does not support it. To add to this issue, a study from the Johns Hopkins Hospital found no evidence that margin positivity (LGD or HGD) was associated with recurrence anywhere in the gland [78]. The discordance in the literature is likely a result of underpowered analyses assessing an incidence that occurs with a low frequency. Further, this entire discussion rests heavily on the premise that an expert pathologist is present to assess the margins during intraoperative consultation (frozen section); such assessment presents great challenges, including differentiating hyperplasia from neoplasia, and interpreting the significance of a margin that only shows denuded epithelium and inflammation, which may be an indication of an adjacent tumor [10].

## Follow-up of Non-Resected Patients

The surveillance of patients with non-resected BD-IPMN is a contentious issue, which continues to spur debate among experts in the field. Advocates for continued surveillance base their arguments not only upon the potential for progression within IPMN but also upon the risk of developing concomitant PDAC elsewhere in the gland [79, 80]. Initial patient assessment should include investigation with dual-phase pancreatic protocol CT and MRI or MRCP; whether to additionally perform EUS depends on the presence of symptoms and cyst characteristics. As we discussed previously, analysis of the different components of the cyst fluid remains a highly complex exercise and, if performed, it should ideally take place in centers with extensive experience caring for patients with this disease and its results should be interpreted with caution. The independent value of circulating markers (e.g. serum CA 19-9, blood NLR) remains to be confirmed, and the inclusion of elevated serum CA 19-9 as a worrisome feature in the revised IAP 2012 Fukuoka consensus guidelines will likely motivate validation studies of its utility.

There is no firm evidence to guide the periodicity or the duration of surveillance after deciding that a patient does not meet the criteria for resection. Retrospective studies have provided important clues on this issue, but ultimately, long-term prospective series will be necessary to answer this question more decisively. Current IAP guidelines use cyst size and growth as the main pacemakers for surveillance periodicity [10]. For cysts less than 2 cm in size, they recommend imaging with CT or MRI every 6 months, which may be spaced out to every 2 years if there are no changes. In patients with cysts >2 cm, more frequent evaluation with EUS (every 3–6 months) is recommended early on, followed by annual surveillance alternating EUS with MRI; these patients represent a tremendous challenge, especially young individuals with long life expectancy for whom the risk of pancreatic resection must be weighed against the financial and emotional cost of continued surveillance. The AGA guidelines [11] are much less granular regarding patient surveillance, recommending evaluation every 2 years regardless of the size of the cyst. Our surveillance strategy at MGH consists of evaluation every 6 months for the first year, then annually for the next 3 years if there is no evidence of cyst growth or development of new features (e.g. mural nodules, wall thickening), and then every 2 years.

The growing number of asymptomatic pancreatic cysts being diagnosed has placed a strong emphasis on the duration of follow-up of patients not undergoing surgery. The AGA guidelines recommend discontinuation of surveillance after 5 years of initial diagnosis if there are no significant changes in the cyst. Our experience demonstrates that this is not a safe strategy, with cases of invasive carcinoma arising from IPMN after 10 years of initial diagnosis [17, 81]. In a series of 577 patients with suspected or presumed BD-IPMN under surveillance at MGH, we recently showed that risk of pancreatic malignancy (defined in this study as HGD or invasive carcinoma arising from IPMN, or concomitant PDAC) does not normalize after 5 years [17]. Among patients who were followed for more than 5 years, pancreatic malignancy developed in 5.5% as well as in 4.1% of those followed for more than 10 years. Notably, among patients who reached 5 years of follow-up without developing worrisome features, the age-standardized risk of pancreatic malignancy was 18.8-fold (95% CI 9.7–32.8; $p < 0.001$) higher compared to that of the US general population. Thus, we strongly advocate for continued surveillance of patients eligible for surgery after 5 years of the initial diagnosis. Last, this study also allowed us to identify a subgroup of patients in whom the risk of pancreatic malignancy is very low and who may be candidates for limited surveillance. We observed that among patients whose cysts remained equal or smaller than 1.5 cm throughout 5 years, only one case of pancreatic malignancy developed, and it was a concomitant PDAC away from the cyst.

## IAP and AGA Guidelines: How We Use Them

The IAP consensus guidelines have evolved substantially since their first edition in 2006 [8]. The IAP Sendai consensus guidelines recommended surgical resection for i) all patients with MD-IPMN and ii) patients with BD-IPMN demonstrating either a) clinical symptoms, b) cysts ≥3 cm in size, or c) mural nodules. These guidelines proved to be very safe in terms of invasive carcinoma (most series reported that practically no cases were missed if these guidelines were followed), while missing approximately 6.5% of patients with HDG [29, 47]. However, evidence suggesting that adherence to these guidelines resulted in overtreatment (patients undergoing surgery for BD-IPMN not showing HGD or invasive carcinoma [82]) led to the IAP 2012 Fukuoka consensus guidelines, which took a more conservative stance. The Fukuoka guidelines de-emphasized the importance of cyst size, which now is no longer an indication for resection by itself, and introduced two layers of risk stratification: worrisome features and high-risk stigmata [9]. Worrisome features include acute pancreatitis, size >3 cm, thickened/enhancing cyst walls, MPD size 5–9 mm, non-enhancing mural nodules, lymphadenopathy, and abrupt change in MPD caliber with distal pancreatic atrophy. Patients with any of these characteristics should undergo EUS and obtain cytology, and if the latter is positive, resection is recommended; if negative or inconclusive, then close surveillance with CT/MRI or EUS is warranted. Presence of high-risk stigmata, namely obstructive jaundice, an enhancing mural nodule, and MPD ≥10 mm, is an indication for resection in surgically fit patients. The utility and accuracy of these new guidelines have been validated [49, 83], but our experience suggests that they may be too conservative. In a series of 563 patients with BD-IPMN undergoing resection or under surveillance at MGH, we found that removing the 3 cm size threshold doubled the number of missed cases with HGD and would have led to one missed case of invasive carcinoma [29]. As mentioned earlier, we do not know the natural history of lesions with HGD, but the stakes are too high when dealing with pancreatic cancer. Thus, while at MGH we have largely followed the different versions of the IAP consensus guidelines, we recommend that the IAP 2012 Fukuoka consensus guidelines (and its recent revision) be used cautiously, especially in young patients with long life expectancy. Expectedly, not all validation studies have agreed with the IAP consensus guidelines. Two studies – one from the University of Heidelberg and another from the H. Lee Moffitt Cancer Center – have reported that the combined risk of HGD or invasive carcinoma in BD-IPMN is 25–57% for sub-centimeter cysts and 26–28% for cysts 1–2 cm in size [84, 85]. These figures are perplexing, especially if we keep in mind that some 10% of individuals older than 70 years have a sub-centimeter pancreatic cyst. Our own experience and reports by other groups lead us to believe that this seemingly high prevalence of HGD and invasive carcinoma arising from very small BD-IPMN could be explained by the presence of a small IPMN with LGD adjacent to a concomitant conventional PDAC, as the distinction between the two events is often challenging [10, 74, 75].

The AGA guidelines put forth in 2015 have marked differences from any edition of the IAP consensus guidelines and from our institutional posture [11]. Among their 10 recommendations, the main difference in terms of determining who should undergo surgery is that resection is recommended only for patients with two of three concerning features (namely, size >3 cm, a mural nodule, or MPD dilation) *and* with evidence of malignancy after EUS; at the same time, the authors recognize that the sensitivity of EUS-guided cytological analysis is only 60%, which means that 40% of patients with cancer will be missed if we applied these criteria. Another critical departure from our practice is the recommendation to stop patient surveillance after IPMN resection. This point came as a shock to many surgeons who have cared for patients with IPMN in whom an invasive recurrence occurs as many as 11 years after primary resection [69] and runs contrary to current evidence on the risk of recurrence of IPMN and of concomitant PDAC. Last, as discussed in the previous section, the recommendation to discontinue follow-up of patients with non-resected IPMN after 5 years in the absence of cyst changes is not supported by evidence and is the most critical point where our perspective is not aligned with the AGA guidelines.

## Conclusions

In summary, IPMN represents a precursor to pancreatic cancer that offers a unique window of opportunity to intervene and impact the historically poor prognosis of the disease. However, overutilization of surgery may result in unnecessary morbidity and mortality and should be tailored to the individual patient's risk of developing cancer. In our opinion, the 2012 IAP Fukuoka consensus guidelines are safe with the caveat that they should be exercised with caution in younger patients. Radiographic surveillance should be continued after resection of worrisome lesions given the continued risk of recurrence or development of metachronous lesions. Future studies should focus on the development of fluid and serum biomarkers that can more accurately identify lesions with HGD in the preoperative setting, which will allow for better risk stratification of IPMN.

## Disclosure Statement

The authors have no conflicts of interest to disclose.

## References

1 Valsangkar NP, Morales-Oyarvide V, Thayer SP, Ferrone CR, Wargo JA, Warshaw AL, Fernandez-del Castillo C: 851 resected cystic tumors of the pancreas: a 33-year experience at the Massachusetts General Hospital. Surgery 2012;152:S4–12.
2 Basturk O, Hong SM, Wood LD, et al.; Baltimore Consensus Meeting: A revised classification system and recommendations from the Baltimore consensus meeting for neoplastic precursor lesions in the pancreas. Am J Surg Pathol 2015;39:1730–1741.
3 Mino-Kenudson M, Fernandez-del Castillo C, Baba Y, Valsangkar NP, Liss AS, Hsu M, Correa-Gallego C, Ingkakul T, Perez Johnston R, Turner BG, Androutsopoulos V, Deshpande V, McGrath D, Sahani DV, Brugge WR, Ogino S, Pitman MB, Warshaw AL, Thayer SP: Prognosis of invasive intraductal papillary mucinous neoplasm depends on histological and precursor epithelial subtypes. Gut 2011;60:1712–1720.
4 Furukawa T, Hatori T, Fujita I, Yamamoto M, Kobayashi M, Ohike N, Morohoshi T, Egawa S, Unno M, Takao S, Osako M, Yonezawa S, Mino-Kenudson M, Lauwers GY, Yamaguchi H, Ban S, Shimizu M: Prognostic relevance of morphological types of intraductal papillary mucinous neoplasms of the pancreas. Gut 2011;60:509–516.
5 Wu J, Matthaei H, Maitra A, Dal Molin M, Wood LD, Eshleman JR, Goggins M, Canto MI, Schulick RD, Edil BH, Wolfgang CL, Klein AP, Diaz LA Jr, Allen PJ, Schmidt CM, Kinzler KW, Papadopoulos N, Hruban RH, Vogelstein B: Recurrent GNAS mutations define an unexpected pathway for pancreatic cyst development. Sci Transl Med 2011;3:92ra66.
6 Furukawa T, Kuboki Y, Tanji E, Yoshida S, Hatori T, Yamamoto M, Shibata N, Shimizu K, Kamatani N, Shiratori K: Whole-exome sequencing uncovers frequent GNAS mutations in intraductal papillary mucinous neoplasms of the pancreas. Sci Rep 2011;1:161.
7 Tamura K, Ohtsuka T, Date K, Fujimoto T, Matsunaga T, Kimura H, Watanabe Y, Miyazaki T, Ohuchida K, Takahata S, Ishigami K, Oda Y, Mizumoto K, Nakamura M, Tanaka M: Distinction of invasive carcinoma derived from intraductal papillary mucinous neoplasms from concomitant ductal adenocarcinoma of the pancreas using molecular biomarkers. Pancreas 2016;45:826–835.
8 Tanaka M, Chari S, Adsay V, Fernandez-del Castillo C, Falconi M, Shimizu M, Yamaguchi K, Yamao K, Matsuno S; International Association of Pancreatology: International consensus guidelines for management of intraductal papillary mucinous neoplasms and mucinous cystic neoplasms of the pancreas. Pancreatology 2006;6:17–32.

9 Tanaka M, Fernandez-del Castillo C, Adsay V, Chari S, Falconi M, Jang JY, Kimura W, Levy P, Pitman MB, Schmidt CM, Shimizu M, Wolfgang CL, Yamaguchi K, Yamao K; International Association of Pancreatology: International consensus guidelines 2012 for the management of IPMN and MCN of the pancreas. Pancreatology 2012;12:183–197.
10 Tanaka M, Fernandez-del Castillo C, Kamisawa T, Jang JY, Levy P, Ohtsuka T, Salvia R, Shimizu Y, Tada M, Wolfgang CL: Revisions of international consensus Fukuoka guidelines for the management of IPMN of the pancreas. Pancreatology 2017;17:738–753.
11 Vege SS, Ziring B, Jain R, Moayyedi P; Clinical Guidelines Committee; American Gastroenterology Association: American Gastroenterological Association Institute guideline on the diagnosis and management of asymptomatic neoplastic pancreatic cysts. Gastroenterology 2015;148:819–822.
12 Scheiman JM, Hwang JH, Moayyedi P: American Gastroenterological Association technical review on the diagnosis and management of asymptomatic neoplastic pancreatic cysts. Gastroenterology 2015;148:824–848.e822.
13 Laffan TA, Horton KM, Klein AP, Berlanstein B, Siegelman SS, Kawamoto S, Johnson PT, Fishman EK, Hruban RH: Prevalence of unsuspected pancreatic cysts on MDCT. AJR Am J Roentgenol 2008;191:802–807.
14 Zhang XM, Mitchell DG, Dohke M, Holland GA, Parker L: Pancreatic cysts: depiction on single-shot fast spin-echo MR images. Radiology 2002;223:547–553.
15 Fernandez-del Castillo C, Targarona J, Thayer SP, Rattner DW, Brugge WR, Warshaw AL: Incidental pancreatic cysts: clinicopathologic characteristics and comparison with symptomatic patients. Arch Surg 2003;138:427–433; discussion 433–434.
16 de Jong K, Nio CY, Hermans JJ, Dijkgraaf MG, Gouma DJ, van Eijck CH, van Heel E, Klass G, Fockens P, Bruno MJ: High prevalence of pancreatic cysts detected by screening magnetic resonance imaging examinations. Clin Gastroenterol Hepatol 2010;8:806–811.
17 Pergolini I, Sahora K, Ferrone CR, Morales-Oyarvide V, Wolpin BM, Mucci LA, Brugge WR, Mino-Kenudson M, Patino M, Sahani DV, Warshaw AL, Lillemoe KD, Fernandez-del Castillo C: Long-term risk of pancreatic malignancy in patients with branch duct intraductal papillary mucinous neoplasm in a referral center. Gastroenterology 2017;153:1284–1294.e1.
18 Waters JA, Schmidt CM, Pinchot JW, White PB, Cummings OW, Pitt HA, Sandrasegaran K, Akisik F, Howard TJ, Nakeeb A, Zyromski NJ, Lillemoe KD: CT vs MRCP: optimal classification of IPMN type and extent. J Gastrointest Surg 2008;12:101–109.
19 Baiocchi GL, Portolani N, Missale G, Baronchelli C, Gheza F, Cantu M, Grazioli L, Giulini SM: Intraductal papillary mucinous neoplasm of the pancreas (IPMN): clinico-pathological correlations and surgical indications. World J Surg Oncol 2010;8:25.
20 Sahora K, Fernandez-del Castillo C, Dong F, Marchegiani G, Thayer SP, Ferrone CR, Sahani DV, Brugge WR, Warshaw AL, Lillemoe KD, Mino-Kenudson M: Not all mixed-type intraductal papillary mucinous neoplasms behave like main-duct lesions: implications of minimal involvement of the main pancreatic duct. Surgery 2014;156:611–621.
21 Morales-Oyarvide V, Pergolini I, Ferrone CR, Mino-Kenudson M, Warshaw AL, Lillemoe KD, Fernandez-del Castillo C: Main pancreatic duct size independently predicts histological main duct involvement, intestinal phenotype, and malignancy in intraductal papillary mucinous neoplasm. Pancreas 2016;45:1526.
22 Adsay NV, Kloppel G, Fukushima N: Intraductal neoplasms of the pancreas; in Bosman FT, Carneiro F, Hruban RH, Theise ND (eds): WHO Classification of Tumors. Lyon, WHO Press, 2010, pp 304–313.
23 Adsay V, Mino-Kenudson M, Furukawa T, et al.; Members of Verona Consensus Meeting, 2013: Pathologic evaluation and reporting of intraductal papillary mucinous neoplasms of the pancreas and other tumoral intraepithelial neoplasms of pancreatobiliary tract: recommendations of Verona consensus meeting. Ann Surg 2016;263:162–177.
24 Adsay NV, Merati K, Basturk O, Iacobuzio-Donahue C, Levi E, Cheng JD, Sarkar FH, Hruban RH, Klimstra DS: Pathologically and biologically distinct types of epithelium in intraductal papillary mucinous neoplasms: delineation of an 'intestinal' pathway of carcinogenesis in the pancreas. Am J Surg Pathol 2004;28: 839–848.
25 Mohri D, Asaoka Y, Ijichi H, Miyabayashi K, Kudo Y, Seto M, Ohta M, Tada M, Tanaka Y, Ikenoue T, Tateishi K, Isayama H, Kanai F, Fukushima N, Tada M, Kawabe T, Omata M, Koike K: Different subtypes of intraductal papillary mucinous neoplasm in the pancreas have distinct pathways to pancreatic cancer progression. J Gastroenterol 2012;47:203–213.
26 Tan MC, Basturk O, Brannon AR, Bhanot U, Scott SN, Bouvier N, LaFemina J, Jarnagin WR, Berger MF, Klimstra D, Allen PJ: GNAS and KRAS mutations define separate progression pathways in intraductal papillary mucinous neoplasm-associated carcinoma. J Am Coll Surg 2015;220:845–854.e841.
27 Marchegiani G, Mino-Kenudson M, Ferrone CR, Warshaw AL, Lillemoe KD, Fernandez-del Castillo C: Oncocytic-type intraductal papillary mucinous neoplasms: a unique malignant pancreatic tumor with good long-term prognosis. J Am Coll Surg 2015;220:839–844.
28 Morales-Oyarvide V, Mino-Kenudson M, Ferrone C, Warshaw AL, Lillemoe KD, Sahani DV, Pergolini I, Attiyeh M, Al Efishat M, Rezaee N, Hruban RH, He J, Weiss MJ, Allen PJ, Wolfgang CL, Fernandez-del Castillo C: Intraductal papillary mucinous neoplasm of the pancreas in young patients: tumor biology, clinical features, and survival outcomes. J Gastrointest Surg 2017;DOI: 10.1007/s11605-017-3602-z.
29 Sahora K, Mino-Kenudson M, Brugge W, Thayer SP, Ferrone CR, Sahani D, Pitman MB, Warshaw AL, Lillemoe KD, Fernandez-del Castillo C: Branch duct intraductal papillary mucinous neoplasms: does cyst size change the tip of the scale? A critical analysis of the revised international consensus guidelines in a large single-institutional series. Ann Surg 2013;258:466–475.
30 Pannala R, Leirness JB, Bamlet WR, Basu A, Petersen GM, Chari ST: Prevalence and clinical profile of pancreatic cancer-associated diabetes mellitus. Gastroenterology 2008;134:981–987.
31 Morales-Oyarvide V, Mino-Kenudson M, Ferrone CR, Sahani DV, Pergolini I, Negreros-Osuna AA, Warshaw AL, Lillemoe KD, Fernandez-del Castillo C: Diabetes mellitus in intraductal papillary mucinous neoplasm of the pancreas is associated with high-grade dysplasia and invasive carcinoma. Pancreatology 2017;17:920–926.
32 Morales-Oyarvide V, Mino-Kenudson M, Ferrone CR, Gonzalez-Gonzalez LA, Warshaw AL, Lillemoe KD, Fernandez-del Castillo C: Acute pancreatitis in intraductal papillary mucinous neoplasms: a common predictor of malignant intestinal subtype. Surgery 2015; 158:1219–1225.
33 Ferrone CR, Finkelstein DM, Thayer SP, Muzikansky A, Fernandez-del Castillo C, Warshaw AL: Perioperative CA19-9 levels can predict stage and survival in patients with resectable pancreatic adenocarcinoma. J Clin Oncol 2006;24:2897–2902.
34 Wang W, Zhang L, Chen L, Wei J, Sun Q, Xie Q, Zhou X, Zhou D, Huang P, Yang Q, Xie H, Zhou L, Zheng S: Serum carcinoembryonic antigen and carbohydrate antigen 19-9 for prediction of malignancy and invasiveness in intraductal papillary mucinous neoplasms of the pancreas: a meta-analysis. Biomed Rep 2015;3:43–50.
35 Morales-Oyarvide V, Mino-Kenudson M, Ferrone CR, Warshaw AL, Lillemoe KD, Fernandez-del Castillo C: Su1353 elevated serum CA19-9 in IPMN is a highly-specific marker of invasive cancer and an independent predictor of advanced stage and poor survival. Gastroenterology 2016;150:S501.
36 Kim JR, Jang JY, Kang MJ, Park T, Lee SY, Jung W, Chang J, Shin Y, Han Y, Kim SW: Clinical implication of serum carcinoembryonic antigen and carbohydrate antigen 19-9 for the prediction of malignancy in intraductal papillary mucinous neoplasm of pancreas. J Hepatobiliary Pancreat Sci 2015;22:699–707.
37 Fritz S, Hackert T, Hinz U, Hartwig W, Buchler MW, Werner J: Role of serum carbohydrate antigen 19-9 and carcinoembryonic antigen in distinguishing between benign and invasive intraductal papillary mucinous neoplasm of the pancreas. Br J Surg 2011;98:104–110.
38 Arima K, Okabe H, Hashimoto D, Chikamoto A, Kuroki H, Taki K, Kaida T, Higashi T, Nitta H, Komohara Y, Beppu T, Takeya M, Baba H: The neutrophil-to-lymphocyte ratio predicts malignant potential in intraductal papillary mucinous neoplasms. J Gastrointest Surg 2015;19:2171–2177.
39 Gemenetzis G, Bagante F, Griffin JF, Rezaee N, Javed AA, Manos LL, Lennon AM, Wood LD, Hruban RH, Zheng L, Zaheer A, Fishman EK, Ahuja N, Cameron JL, Weiss MJ, He J, Wolfgang CL: Neutrophil-to-lymphocyte ratio is a predictive marker for invasive malignancy in intraductal papillary mucinous neoplasms of the pancreas. Ann Surg 2017;266:339–345.
40 Sainani NI, Saokar A, Deshpande V, Fernandez-del Castillo C, Hahn P, Sahani DV: Comparative performance of MDCT and MRI with MR cholangiopancreatography in characterizing small pancreatic cysts. AJR Am J Roentgenol 2009;193:722–731.
41 Sahani DV, Sainani NI, Blake MA, Crippa S, Mino-Kenudson M, Fernandez-del Castillo C: Prospective evaluation of reader performance on MDCT in characterization of cystic pancreatic lesions and prediction of cyst biologic aggressiveness. AJR Am J Roentgenol 2011;197:W53–61.
42 Hirono S, Tani M, Kawai M, Okada K, Miyazawa M, Shimizu A, Kitahata Y, Yamaue H: The carcinoembryonic antigen level in pancreatic juice and mural nodule size are predictors of malignancy for branch duct type intraductal papillary mucinous neoplasms of the pancreas. Ann Surg 2012;255:517–522.
43 Ohno E, Itoh A, Kawashima H, Ishikawa T, Matsubara H, Itoh Y, Nakamura Y, Hiramatsu T, Nakamura M, Miyahara R, Ohmiya N, Ishigami M, Katano Y, Goto H, Hirooka Y: Malignant transformation of branch duct-type intraductal papillary mucinous neoplasms of the pancreas based on contrast-enhanced endoscopic ultrasonography morphological changes: focus on malignant transformation of intraductal papillary mucinous neoplasm itself. Pancreas 2012;41:855–862.
44 Seo N, Byun JH, Kim JH, Kim HJ, Lee SS, Song KB, Kim SC, Han DJ, Hong SM, Lee MG: Validation of the 2012 international consensus guidelines using computed tomography and magnetic resonance imaging: branch duct and main duct intraductal papillary mucinous neoplasms of the pancreas. Ann Surg 2016;263:557–564.
45 Berland LL, Silverman SG, Gore RM, Mayo-Smith WW, Megibow AJ, Yee J, Brink JA, Baker ME, Federle MP, Foley WD, Francis IR, Herts BR, Israel GM, Krinsky G, Platt JF, Shuman WP, Taylor AJ: Managing incidental findings on abdominal CT: white paper of the ACR incidental findings committee. J Am Coll Radiol 2010;7:754–773.
46 Salvia R, Fernandez-del Castillo C, Bassi C, Thayer SP, Falconi M, Mantovani W, Pederzoli P, Warshaw AL: Main-duct intraductal papillary mucinous neoplasms of the pancreas: clinical predictors of malignancy and long-term survival following resection. Ann Surg 2004; 239:678–685; discussion 685–687.

47 Fernandez-del Castillo C, Adsay NV: Intraductal papillary mucinous neoplasms of the pancreas. Gastroenterology 2010;139:708–713.

48 Rodriguez JR, Salvia R, Crippa S, Warshaw AL, Bassi C, Falconi M, Thayer SP, Lauwers GY, Capelli P, Mino-Kenudson M, Razo O, McGrath D, Pederzoli P, Fernandez-del Castillo C: Branch-duct intraductal papillary mucinous neoplasms: observations in 145 patients who underwent resection. Gastroenterology 2007;133:72–79.

49 Kim KW, Park SH, Pyo J, Yoon SH, Byun JH, Lee MG, Krajewski KM, Ramaiya NH: Imaging features to distinguish malignant and benign branch-duct type intraductal papillary mucinous neoplasms of the pancreas: a meta-analysis. Ann Surg 2014;259:72–81.

50 Anand N, Sampath K, Wu BU: Cyst features and risk of malignancy in intraductal papillary mucinous neoplasms of the pancreas: a meta-analysis. Clin Gastroenterol Hepatol 2013;11:913–921.

51 Kitano M, Sakamoto H, Komaki T, Kudo M: New techniques and future perspective of EUS for the differential diagnosis of pancreatic malignancies: contrast harmonic imaging. Dig Endosc 2011;23(suppl 1):46–50.

52 Correa-Gallego C, Warshaw AL, Fernandez-del Castillo C: Fluid CEA in IPMNs: a useful test or the flip of a coin? Am J Gastroenterol 2009;104:796–797.

53 Brugge WR, Lewandrowski K, Lee-Lewandrowski E, Centeno BA, Szydlo T, Regan S, Fernandez-del Castillo C, Warshaw AL: Diagnosis of pancreatic cystic neoplasms: a report of the cooperative pancreatic cyst study. Gastroenterology 2004;126:1330–1336.

54 Cizginer S, Turner BG, Bilge AR, Karaca C, Pitman MB, Brugge WR: Cyst fluid carcinoembryonic antigen is an accurate diagnostic marker of pancreatic mucinous cysts. Pancreas 2011;40:1024–1028.

55 Das KK, Xiao H, Geng X, Fernandez-del Castillo C, Morales-Oyarvide V, Daglilar E, Forcione DG, Bounds BC, Brugge WR, Pitman MB, Mino-Kenudson M, Das KM: mAb Das-1 is specific for high-risk and malignant intraductal papillary mucinous neoplasm (IPMN). Gut 2014;63:1626–1634.

56 Das KK, Geng XG, Morales-Oyarvide V, Huynh T, Pergolini I, Pitman MB, Ferrone C, Brugge W, Al Efishat M, Haviland D, Thompson E, Wolfgang C, Lennon AM, Allen P, Lillemoe KD, Fernandez-del Castillo C, Das KM, Mino-Kenudson M: 666 – A multicenter, validation study of cyst fluid analysis for mAb-Das1 for the identification of high-risk and malignant mucinous cysts of the pancreas. Gastroenterology 2017;152:S146–S147.

57 Pitman MB, Genevay M, Yaeger K, Chebib I, Turner BG, Mino-Kenudson M, Brugge WR: High-grade atypical epithelial cells in pancreatic mucinous cysts are a more accurate predictor of malignancy than 'positive' cytology. Cancer Cytopathol 2010;118:434–440.

58 Pitman MB, Yaeger KA, Brugge WR, Mino-Kenudson M: Prospective analysis of atypical epithelial cells as a high-risk cytologic feature for malignancy in pancreatic cysts. Cancer Cytopathol 2013;121:29–36.

59 Fritz S, Fernandez-del Castillo C, Mino-Kenudson M, Crippa S, Deshpande V, Lauwers GY, Warshaw AL, Thayer SP, Iafrate AJ: Global genomic analysis of intraductal papillary mucinous neoplasms of the pancreas reveals significant molecular differences compared to ductal adenocarcinoma. Ann Surg 2009;249:440–447.

60 Jones M, Zheng Z, Wang J, Dudley J, Albanese E, Kadayifci A, Dias-Santagata D, Le L, Brugge WR, Fernandez-del Castillo C, Mino-Kenudson M, Iafrate AJ, Pitman MB: Impact of next-generation sequencing on the clinical diagnosis of pancreatic cysts. Gastrointest Endosc 2016;83:140–148.

61 Springer S, Wang Y, Dal Molin M, et al: A combination of molecular markers and clinical features improve the classification of pancreatic cysts. Gastroenterology 2015;149:1501–1510.

62 Crippa S, Fernandez-del Castillo C, Salvia R, Finkelstein D, Bassi C, Dominguez I, Muzikansky A, Thayer SP, Falconi M, Mino-Kenudson M, Capelli P, Lauwers GY, Partelli S, Pederzoli P, Warshaw AL: Mucin-producing neoplasms of the pancreas: an analysis of distinguishing clinical and epidemiologic characteristics. Clin Gastroenterol Hepatol 2010;8:213–219.

63 Fernandez-del Castillo C, Morales-Oyarvide V, McGrath D, Wargo JA, Ferrone CR, Thayer SP, Lillemoe KD, Warshaw AL: Evolution of the Whipple procedure at the Massachusetts General Hospital. Surgery 2012;152:S56–63.

64 Fong ZV, Alvino DM, Fernandez-del Castillo C, Nipp RD, Traeger LN, Ruddy M, Lubitz CC, Johnson CD, Chang DC, Warshaw AL, Lillemoe KD, Ferrone CR: Health-related quality of life and functional outcomes in 5-year survivors after pancreaticoduodenectomy. Ann Surg 2017;266:685–692.

65 Sahora K, Ferrone CR, Brugge WR, Morales-Oyarvide V, Warshaw AL, Lillemoe KD, Fernandez-del Castillo C: Effects of comorbidities on outcomes of patients with intraductal papillary mucinous neoplasms. Clin Gastroenterol Hepatol 2015;13:1816–1823.

66 Sauvanet A, Gaujoux S, Blanc B, Couvelard A, Dokmak S, Vullierme MP, Ruszniewski P, Belghiti J, Levy P: Parenchyma-sparing pancreatectomy for presumed noninvasive intraductal papillary mucinous neoplasms of the pancreas. Ann Surg 2014;260:364–371.

67 Faitot F, Gaujoux S, Barbier L, Novaes M, Dokmak S, Aussilhou B, Couvelard A, Rebours V, Ruszniewski P, Belghiti J, Sauvanet A: Reappraisal of pancreatic enucleations: a single-center experience of 126 procedures. Surgery 2015;158:201–210.

68 Kaiser J, Fritz S, Klauss M, Bergmann F, Hinz U, Strobel O, Schneider L, Buchler MW, Hackert T: Enucleation: a treatment alternative for branch duct intraductal papillary mucinous neoplasms. Surgery 2017; 161:602–610.

69 Marchegiani G, Mino-Kenudson M, Ferrone CR, Morales-Oyarvide V, Warshaw AL, Lillemoe KD, Fernandez-del Castillo C: Patterns of recurrence after resection of IPMN: who, when, and how? Ann Surg 2015; 262:1108–1114.

70 Kang MJ, Jang JY, Lee KB, Chang YR, Kwon W, Kim SW: Long-term prospective cohort study of patients undergoing pancreatectomy for intraductal papillary mucinous neoplasm of the pancreas: implications for postoperative surveillance. Ann Surg 2014;260:356–363.

71 White R, D'Angelica M, Katabi N, Tang L, Klimstra D, Fong Y, Brennan M, Allen P: Fate of the remnant pancreas after resection of noninvasive intraductal papillary mucinous neoplasm. J Am Coll Surg 2007;204: 987–993; discussion 993–995.

72 Salvia R, Partelli S, Crippa S, Landoni L, Capelli P, Manfredi R, Bassi C, Pederzoli P: Intraductal papillary mucinous neoplasms of the pancreas with multifocal involvement of branch ducts. Am J Surg 2009;198:709–714.

73 Marchegiani G, Mino-Kenudson M, Sahora K, Morales-Oyarvide V, Thayer S, Ferrone C, Warshaw AL, Lillemoe KD, Fernandez-del Castillo C: IPMN involving the main pancreatic duct: biology, epidemiology, and long-term outcomes following resection. Ann Surg 2015;261:976–983.

74 Ingkakul T, Sadakari Y, Ienaga J, Satoh N, Takahata S, Tanaka M: Predictors of the presence of concomitant invasive ductal carcinoma in intraductal papillary mucinous neoplasm of the pancreas. Ann Surg 2010;251: 70–75.

75 Ideno N, Ohtsuka T, Kono H, Fujiwara K, Oda Y, Aishima S, Ito T, Ishigami K, Tokunaga S, Ohuchida K, Takahata S, Nakamura M, Mizumoto K, Tanaka M: Intraductal papillary mucinous neoplasms of the pancreas with distinct pancreatic ductal adenocarcinomas are frequently of gastric subtype. Ann Surg 2013;258: 141–151.

76 Miyasaka Y, Ohtsuka T, Tamura K, Mori Y, Shindo K, Yamada D, Takahata S, Ishigami K, Ito T, Tokunaga S, Oda Y, Mizumoto K, Nakamura M, Tanaka M: Predictive factors for the metachronous development of high-risk lesions in the remnant pancreas after partial pancreatectomy for intraductal papillary mucinous neoplasm. Ann Surg 2016;263:1180–1187.

77 Frankel TL, LaFemina J, Bamboat ZM, D'Angelica MI, DeMatteo RP, Fong Y, Kingham TP, Jarnagin WR, Allen PJ: Dysplasia at the surgical margin is associated with recurrence after resection of non-invasive intraductal papillary mucinous neoplasms. HPB (Oxford) 2013;15:814–821.

78 He J, Cameron JL, Ahuja N, Makary MA, Hirose K, Choti MA, Schulick RD, Hruban RH, Pawlik TM, Wolfgang CL: Is it necessary to follow patients after resection of a benign pancreatic intraductal papillary mucinous neoplasm? J Am Coll Surg 2013;216:657–665.

79 Ohtsuka T, Kono H, Tanabe R, Nagayoshi Y, Mori Y, Sadakari Y, Takahata S, Oda Y, Aishima S, Igarashi H, Ito T, Ishigami K, Nakamura M, Mizumoto K, Tanaka M: Follow-up study after resection of intraductal papillary mucinous neoplasm of the pancreas; special references to the multifocal lesions and development of ductal carcinoma in the remnant pancreas. Am J Surg 2012;204:44–48.

80 Tanno S, Nakano Y, Sugiyama Y, Nakamura K, Sasajima J, Koizumi K, Yamazaki M, Nishikawa T, Mizukami Y, Yanagawa N, Fujii T, Obara T, Okumura T, Kohgo Y: Incidence of synchronous and metachronous pancreatic carcinoma in 168 patients with branch duct intraductal papillary mucinous neoplasm. Pancreatology 2010;10:173–178.

81 Honselmann KC, Patino M, Mino-Kenudson M, Ferrone C, Warshaw AL, Fernandez-del Castillo C, Lillemoe KD: Ductal carcinoma arising in a largely unchanged presumed branch-duct IPMN after 10 years of surveillance. Ann Surg 2017;266:e38–e40.

82 Pelaez-Luna M, Chari ST, Smyrk TC, Takahashi N, Clain JE, Levy MJ, Pearson RK, Petersen BT, Topazian MD, Vege SS, Kendrick M, Farnell MB: Do consensus indications for resection in branch duct intraductal papillary mucinous neoplasm predict malignancy? A study of 147 patients. Am J Gastroenterol 2007;102: 1759–1764.

83 Goh BK, Tan DM, Thng CH, Lee SY, Low AS, Chan CY, Wong JS, Lee VT, Cheow PC, Chow PK, Chung AY, Wong WK, Ooi LL: Are the Sendai and Fukuoka consensus guidelines for cystic mucinous neoplasms of the pancreas useful in the initial triage of all suspected pancreatic cystic neoplasms? A single-institution experience with 317 surgically-treated patients. Ann Surg Oncol 2014;21:1919–1926.

84 Fritz S, Klauss M, Bergmann F, Hackert T, Hartwig W, Strobel O, Bundy BD, Buchler MW, Werner J: Small (Sendai negative) branch-duct IPMNs: not harmless. Ann Surg 2012;256:313–320.

85 Wong J, Weber J, Centeno BA, Vignesh S, Harris CL, Klapman JB, Hodul P: High-grade dysplasia and adenocarcinoma are frequent in side-branch intraductal papillary mucinous neoplasm measuring less than 3 cm on endoscopic ultrasound. J Gastrointest Surg 2013;17:78–84; discussion 84–85.

## Mit Adalimumab Therapieziele erreichen

*In der Therapie der mittelschweren bis schweren aktiven Colitis ulcerosa hat sich Adalimumab (Humira®) in mehr als 5-jähriger klinischer Anwendung bewährt. Aktuelle Real-World-Daten zeigen, dass die antientzündliche Therapie mit dem Tumornekrosefaktor (TNF)-Antagonisten rasch wirksam und sicher ist: Schon früh konnte die Symptomlast reduziert und die Lebensqualität und Zufriedenheit betroffener Patienten verbessert werden. In vielen Fällen konnten eine Remission und Mukosaheilung erreicht und bei guter Verträglichkeit langfristig erhalten werden. Die Adalimumab-Therapie hatte zudem positive Auswirkungen auf die Ressourcen des Gesundheitssystems.*

Die aktuell veröffentlichte InspirADA-Studie untersuchte die Wirksamkeit und Verträglichkeit von Adalimumab im klinischen Alltag. An der internationalen Studie nahmen 463 erwachsene Patienten (18–75 Jahre) mit mittelschwerer bis schwerer aktiver Colitis ulcerosa in 92 Zentren teil [1].

### *Schnelle und deutliche Verbesserung der Symptomatik*

Bereits in Woche 2 der Adalimumab-Therapie erreichten drei Viertel der Patienten (74%) ein klinisches Ansprechen, definiert als eine Abnahme des SCCAI (Simple Clinical Colitis Activity Index) um ≥ 2 Punkte gegenüber Baseline. Die Ansprechrate konnte in Woche 8 auf 79% gesteigert werden. Zum selben Zeitpunkt erzielte etwa die Hälfte der Patienten eine Remission (SCCAI-Wert ≤ 2) (Abb. 1). Diese Ansprech- und Remissionsraten konnten über den gesamten Studienzeitraum aufrechterhalten werden. Auch der Anteil an Patienten mit extraintestinaler Manifestation (EIM, jegliche Form) verringerte sich unter der Anti-TNF-Therapie signifikant von 19% auf 11% (Baseline vs. Woche 26; $p < 0{,}001$) (Abb. 1).

### *Signifikant positiver und anhaltender Effekt auf Lebensqualität und Zufriedenheit*

Die krankheitsbezogene Lebensqualität besserte sich im Studienverlauf signifikant. Indikator hierfür war eine Zunahme des mittleren SIBDQ-Scores (Short Inflammatory Bowel Disease Questionnaire) um 11,1 Punkte in Woche 2 bzw. um 17,4 Punkte in Woche 26 ($p < 0{,}001$). Auch die Zufriedenheit der Patienten mit ihrer Behandlung nahm signifikant zu. Nach 26-wöchiger Therapie wurde für alle Parameter des Treatment Satisfaction Questionnaire for Medication (TSQM) eine Zunahme im Vergleich zu Studienbeginn beobachtet: Wirksamkeit (mittlere Veränderung 24,4), Nebenwirkungen (18,9), Nutzen (6,2) und Gesamtzufriedenheit (22,6) (alle $p < 0{,}001$).

### *Weniger Arbeitsausfälle, mehr Alltagsaktivitäten*

Die Adalimumab-Behandlung hatte einen positiven Effekt auf das Arbeitsleben und die tägliche Aktivität der Betroffenen. So reduzierte sich der Arbeitsausfall um 11%, die Beeinträchtigung während der Arbeit um 24% und die Arbeitsbeeinträchtigung insgesamt um 29% (gemessen am Work Productivity and Activity Impairment (WPAI), Woche 26 vs. Baseline). Überdies nahm die Einschränkung der Patienten bei alltäglichen Aktivitäten signifikant um 27% ab (alle $p < 0{,}001$).

### *Entlastung des Gesundheitssystems*

Die Inanspruchnahme des Gesundheitssystems ging in den 6 Monaten nach Therapiebeginn verglichen mit dem 6-monatigen Zeitraum vor der Studie signifikant zurück. So verringerte sich die mittlere Anzahl der Hospitalisierungen (alle Ursachen und bedingt durch die Colitis ulcerosa) um jeweils 0,3. War eine Krankenhauseinweisung erforderlich, reduzierte sich die Dauer des stationären Aufenthalts signifikant um 3,3 Tage. Auch ambulante Behandlungen waren durch die Adalimumab-Therapie seltener nötig (–4,6) (alle $p < 0{,}001$). Adalimumab wurde gut vertragen und keine neuen Sicherheitssignale wurden beobachtet.

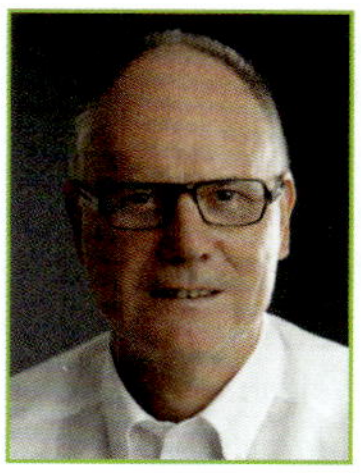

«Aktuelle Real-World-Daten sind für die tägliche Praxis von größerer Bedeutung als Ergebnisse aus klinischen Studien, da sie näher an den realen Bedingungen und Bedürfnissen der Patienten orientiert sind. Für eine erfolgreiche Therapie ist ein gemeinsames Verständnis der Therapieziele erforderlich.
Therapieziele bei der Colitis ulcerosa sind das schnelle Ansprechen im akuten Schub und die langfristige Remissionserhaltung mit der Perspektive einer möglichst normalen Lebensqualität. Hierbei ist für Patienten besonders auch eine schnelle Symptomverbesserung in Bezug auf Blut im Stuhl sowie eine Reduktion der extraintestinalen Manifestationen von Bedeutung.»

*Priv.-Doz. Dr. Bokemeyer, Minden*

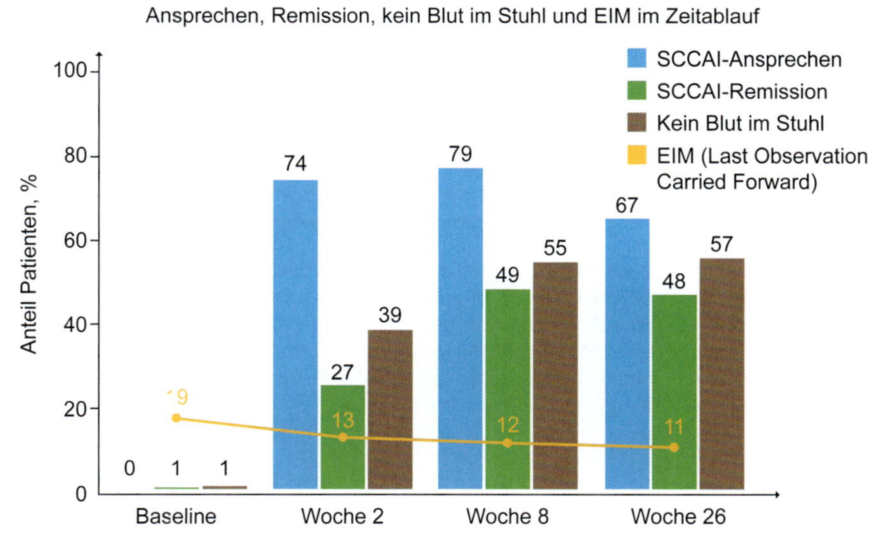


**Abb. 1.** Anteil der Patienten mit Ansprechen und Remission (SCCAI), ohne Blut im Stuhl sowie mit extraintestinaler Manifestation (EIM) unter Adalimumab-Therapie in der InspirADA-Studie im zeitlichen Ablauf, modifiziert nach [2].

### *Literatur*

1 Travis S et al.: J Crohns Colitis 2017;11:1317–1325.
2 Travis S et al.: J Crohns Colitis 2016;10(suppl 1):S391–S392.

Weitere Informationen bei
AbbVie Deutschland GmbH & Co. KG
*www.abbvie.de*

DE/HUG/1217/2931

KARGER

Fax + 49 761 4 52 07 14
Information@Karger.com
www.karger.com

*Aktiver Morbus Crohn*

## Schnell und dauerhaft unter Kontrolle bringen

*Vor einem Jahr wurde der erste Interleukin (IL)-12/23-Inhibitor, Ustekinumab (Stelara®), für die Behandlung erwachsener Patienten mit mittelschwerem bis schwerem Morbus Crohn zugelassen. Ustekinumab zeigt eine schnelle Wirksamkeit, ein gutes Sicherheitsprofil sowie hohe Remissionsraten über einen Beobachtungszeitraum von über 2 Jahren.*

Ustekinumab ist der erste vollständig humanisierte monoklonale Antikörper, der an die p40-Untereinheit von IL-12 und IL-23 bindet – zwei Schlüsselzytokine der Entzündungskaskade des Morbus Crohn [1]. Das Arzneimittel ist seit November 2016 für Patienten mit mittelschwerem bis schwerem aktiven Morbus Crohn zugelassen, die unzureichend oder nicht mehr auf eine konventionelle Therapie oder Tumornekrosefaktor (TNF)-α-Blocker angesprochen haben, diese nicht vertragen haben oder bei denen diese kontraindiziert sind [2]. Mit Ustekinumab steht somit ein neues First-Line-Biologikum zur Verfügung.

*Schnelles Ansprechen bereits nach einer Woche*

Eine aktuelle Post-hoc-Analyse von Patienten, bei denen Anti-TNF-α-Therapien versagt hatten, wies auf signifikante Symptomverbesserungen bereits innerhalb einer Woche nach intravenöser (i.v.) Induktion mit Ustekinumab im Vergleich zu Placebo hin. Die untersuchten Daten basierten auf Patienten-berichteten Crohn's Disease Activity Index (CDAI)-Komponenten wie Stuhlfrequenz, Abdominalschmerz und allgemeines Wohlbefinden der Zulassungsstudie UNITI-1 [3]. Dieses frühe und schnelle Ansprechen wurde auch in den Zulassungsstudien UNITI-1 und -2 belegt: Erste sichtbare Effekte im klinischen Ansprechen zeigten sich dabei bereits nach 3 Wochen. Dabei war das Ansprechen bei Patienten ohne Anti-TNF-α-Versagen höher als bei Patienten mit Anti-TNF-α-Versagen. Den primären Endpunkt (klinisches Ansprechen* nach Woche 6) erreichten in der UNITI-2-Studie signifikant mehr Patienten unter Ustekinumab 6 mg/kg Körpergewicht als unter Placebo (55,5% vs. 28,7%; $p < 0{,}001$) [4]. Dieses Ergebnis könnte richtungsweisend für einen frühen Einsatz von Ustekinumab sein.

*Langanhaltende Remission über 2 Jahre*

Patienten, die in den Induktionsstudien nach 8 Wochen ein klinisches Ansprechen* erreichten, konnten an der Erhaltungsstudie IM-UNITI teilnehmen, die über weitere 44 Wochen lief. Die insgesamt 397 Patienten erhielten anschließend randomisiert 90 mg subkutan (s.c.) Ustekinumab alle 8 Wochen (q8w) oder alle 12 Wochen (q12w)***. Nach 44 Wochen waren 48,8% der Patienten unter Ustekinumab 90 mg s.c. q12w und 53,1% der Patienten unter Ustekinumab 90 mg s.c. q8w in klinischer Remission** (Placebo: 35,9%; $p = 0{,}040$ q12w und $p = 0{,}005$ q8w). Auch die Antikörperbildung ist unter Ustekinumab sehr niedrig: Nach 44 Wochen konnte diese bei lediglich 2,3% der Patienten nachgewiesen werden [4].
Inzwischen stehen Daten über bis zu 2 Jahren zur Verfügung, die eine lang anhaltende Wirksamkeit von Ustekinumab dokumentieren. 298 der 397 Teilnehmer aus IM-UNITI (75%), die bis Woche 44 gut auf Ustekinumab angesprochen hatten, wurden in das Langzeit-Follow-up (long-term extension, LTE) eingeschlossen. Nach Woche 92 waren 79,2% (q12w) und 87,2% (q8w) der Patienten, die Ustekinumab erhielten, in klinischer Remission** [5]. Jeweils 90,9% und 94,3% der Patienten zeigten in Woche 92 ein klinisches Ansprechen* [6]. Bei Patienten, bei denen Ustekinumab frühzeitig eingesetzt wurde (vor einer Anti-TNF-α-Therapie), waren die langfristigen Ansprechraten tendenziell besser. Alle Patienten, die bis Woche 96 mit Ustekinumab behandelt wurden, erreichten Remissions- und Ansprechraten in Woche 92 von jeweils 70,7% bzw. 84,7% (As-observed-Analyse) [5].

*Gute Verträglichkeit*

Ustekinumab erwies sich in den Studien als langfristig gut verträglich: So war die Rate unerwünschter Ereignisse bis Woche 44 in allen Behandlungsgruppen vergleichbar mit Placebo [4]. Auch bis Woche 96 traten keine neuen oder unbekannten Sicherheitssignale auf [5].

* Definiert als eine Reduktion des Baseline Crohn's Disease Activity Index (CDAI)-Scores um mindestens 100 Punkte oder CDAI < 150.
** Definiert als eine Reduktion des CDAI-Scores um mindestens 150 Punkte.
*** Empfohlen wird die Anwendung von Ustekinumab alle 12 Wochen (q12w). Bei unzureichendem Ansprechen 8 Wochen nach der ersten Injektion oder Verlust des Ansprechens bei einer Dosierung alle 12 Wochen kann Ustekinumab alternativ alle 8 Wochen (q8w) verabreicht werden.

*Literatur*

1 Neurath MF et al.: Nat Rev Immunol 2014;14:329–342.
2 Aktuelle Stelara®-Fachinformation 45/90 mg Injektionslösung.
3 Sandborn WJ et al.: WCOG 2017;Poster P2145.
4 Feagan B et al.: N Eng J Med 2016;375:1946–1960.
5 Sandborn WJ et al.: DDW 2017;Poster Su1889.
6 Sandborn WJ et al.: ECCO 2017;abstr OP10.

Weitere Informationen bei
Janssen-Cilag GmbH
*www.janssen.com/germany*

## Bayer wegweisend bei modernen Entwicklungsstandards für die evidenzbasierte Phytotherapie mit Iberogast®

Mit der steigenden Verbrauchernachfrage nach pflanzlichen Arzneimitteln gerät die Gesundheitsindustrie zunehmend in Zugzwang: Sie muss nachweisen, dass pflanzliche Präparate den gleichen Qualitäts-, Sicherheits- und Wirksamkeitsstandards entsprechen wie synthetisch hergestellte Medikamente. Bei der 25. United European Gastroenterology (UEG)-Woche in Barcelona, Spanien, forderte Dr. John O'Mullane, globaler Leiter des Bereichs Innovation und Entwicklung bei der Division Consumer Health von Bayer, deshalb die Branche auf, sich um weltweit anerkannte Standards für die Entwicklung pflanzlicher Produkte zu bemühen. Zusammen mit namhaften Experten auf dem Gebiet der Gastroenterologie legte er die Bedeutung der evidenzbasierten Phytotherapie dar. Im Mittelpunkt stand dabei Iberogast® mit seiner zentralen Bedeutung bei der Behandlung funktioneller Magen-Darm-Störungen. Rund 40% aller Arzneimittel basieren auf pflanzlichen Wirkstoffen [1], und die Weltgesundheitsorganisation schätzt, dass 80% der Menschen bei ihrer medizinischen Grundversorgung auch zu pflanzlichen Arzneimitteln greifen [2]. Die Forschung zeigt, dass Verbraucher verschreibungsfreie pflanzliche Arzneimittel für sicherer als herkömmliche freiverkäufliche Medikamente halten und mindestens für genauso wirksam wie diese [3].

*Literatur*

1 Samuelsson G: Drugs of Natural Origin: A Textbook of Pharmacology, ed 5. Stockholm, Apotekarsocieteten, 2004.
2 World Health Organization (WHO): Self-Care for Health. *www.who.int*, 2014.
3 Kline Market Research Report: Nonprescription Drugs USA. 2017 *https://www.klinegroup.com/reports/cia3.asp* (letzter Aufruf 22.11.2017).

Bayer Vital GmbH
*www.bayer.de*

KARGER

Fax + 49 761 4 52 07 14
Information@Karger.com
www.karger.com

*EndoStim auf dem DGVS-Kongress 2017*

## Zwischenergebnisse zeigen: Neurostimulation ist eine geeignete Therapieoption

Die Therapie der gastroösophagealen Reflux-Krankheit (GERD) mit Protonenpumpen-Inhibitoren (PPI) ist nach wie vor bei etwa 30% der Patienten unzureichend [1]. Die Stimulation des unteren Ösophagussphinkters (lower esopageal sphincter stimulation, LESS) stellt für diese Patienten eine geeignete Option dar, wie Prof. Labenz mit den Zwischenergebnissen des LESS-GERD-Registers [2] zeigen konnte. Der Bedarf an einer neuen Therapieoption wie der Neurostimulation wurde auch in einer interaktiven Falldiskussion betont.

Die prospektive, multizentrische Registerstudie LESS-GERD [2] ist weltweit an 15 Zentren aktiv und wertet EndoStim hinsichtlich seiner Sicherheit in der klinischen Routine aus. Bis dato wurden 215 Patienten in die Studie aufgenommen und bereits 130 Patienten nahmen an einem Follow-up von mindestens 6 Monaten teil, wobei Sicherheitsdaten für alle eingeschlossenen Patienten verfügbar sind.

Die untersuchten Patienten profitierten von der EndoStim-Therapie durch eine verbesserte Lebensqualität mit einer Verbesserung des medianen GERD-HRQL-Scores (HRQL = gesundheitsbezogene Lebensqualität) zu Baseline von 23 auf 8 nach 6 Monaten (gepaarte Daten, n = 110, p < 0,0001). Der mediane Score blieb nach 24 Monaten stabil auf 8 (n = 25). Des Weiteren reduzierte sich der prozentuale Anteil der Patienten mit moderater bis schwerer Regurgitation von 63% (n = 165) zu Baseline auf 13% (n = 67) nach 12 Monaten. Auch die extraösophagealen Symptome und Schlafstörungen konnten unter EndoStim verbessert werden. Der positive Effekt zeigte sich auch bei der Messung der Säureexposition mittels pH-Metrie: Der ösophageale pH < 4,0 über 24 Stunden reduzierte sich von 8,2% zu Baseline auf ein normales Level nach 6 bzw. 12 Monaten (4,1% bzw. 3,6%) [2].

Hinsichtlich Sicherheit und Verträglichkeit zeigte EndoStim folgende Ergebnisse: Die Häufigkeit von Dysphagie und Gasbloat nahm im Laufe von 12 Monaten ab, und es trat lediglich 1 Fall milder postoperativer Dysphagie auf, der ohne Intervention sistiert. Insgesamt traten nur bei 13 von 215 (6%) Patienten schwere unerwünschte Ereignisse auf [2].

Im Rahmen eines Lunch-Symposiums von EndoStim diskutierte ein interdisziplinäres Expertenboard verschiedene Patientenfälle und Herangehensweisen bei GERD mit dem Plenum. Dass die Therapie von GERD zukünftig immer interdisziplinärer betrachtet werden wird, spiegelte sich auch in der Zusammensetzung des Publikums wider: Mit jeweils 46% setzte sich der Großteil der Teilnehmer aus Gastroenterologen und Chirurgen zusammen. Prof. Dr. Ahmed Madisch, Chefarzt für Gastroenterologie im Klinikum Siloah, machte zunächst auf die Unmet Needs von Reflux-Patienten wie nächtliches oder postprandiales Sodbrennen aufmerksam und stellte die Gründe der Patienten für den Wunsch nach einer anderen PPI heraus: unzureichende oder ausbleibende Wirkung, Ablehnung einer dauerhaften Einnahme, Angst vor Nebenwirkungen sowie tatsächliche Nebenwirkungen. Die unzureichende Wirkung von PPI und die unnötig lange Reflux-Beschwerdezeit mahnte auch Prof. Dr. Burkhard von Rahden, Oberarzt der Chirurgischen Klinik Würzburg, an. Beide Experten stützen ihren Bericht mit Patientenfällen, bei denen den Patienten mit EndoStim zu einer guten Symptomkontrolle sowie verbesserter Lebensqualität verholfen werden konnte.

Dass die Anzahl der Sleeve-Gastrektomien in Deutschland stetig ansteigt und in Studien ein postoperativer Anstieg von Reflux zu beobachten war [3], führten Dr. Andreas Grimme, Allgemein- und Viszeralchirurgie Fulda, und Prof. Dr. Bernd Kronenberger, Innere Medizin Fulda, aus. Der postoperative Anstieg von Reflux konnte mit EndoStim effektiv behandelt werden, wie beide Experten anhand eines Patienten vorstellten, der mit EndoStim effektiv behandelt werden konnte.

Ein weiterer Diskussionspunkt war das Verfahren bei Patienten mit familiärer Vorbelastung wie z.B. mit Barrett- oder Ösophaguskarzinom. Als Beispiel stellte Prof. Labenz einen 18-Jährigen vor, der zwar ohne Beschwerden war, aber in der Histologie eine Barrett-Schleimhaut ohne intraepitheliale Neoplasie zeigte. Labenz deutete an, dass in solchen Fällen eine Anti-Reflux-Intervention, wie beispielsweise EndoStim, eine mögliche Option zur Prävention darstellen könnte. Wie anhand der realen Fallbeispiele gezeigt werden konnte, eignet sich EndoStim für die Therapie unterschiedlicher Patiententypen:

- Patienten mit unzureichender Symptomkontrolle unter PPI,
- Patienten nach einer Sleeve-Gastrektomie,
- Patienten, die einen Progress ihrer Erkrankung fürchten.

### Literatur

1 Labenz J et al.: Inadequate symptom control on long-term PPI therapy in GERD – Fact or fiction? (LOPA II study). DDW, May 6–9 2017, Chicago.
2 Labenz J et al.: Z Gastroenterol 2017;55:e72.
3 Laffin M et al.: J Obes 2013;2013:741097.

Weitere Informationen bei
EndoStim BV
*www.endostim.com/de*

## Gilead gibt Phase-II-Ergebnisse für GS-0976 bei nichtalkoholischer Steatohepatitis (NASH) bekannt

Gilead Sciences, Inc. (Nasdaq: GILD) hat Ergebnisse aus einer randomisierten, placebokontrollierten Phase-II-Studie an Patienten mit nichtalkoholischer Steatohepatitis (NASH) bekannt gegeben. Dabei wurden 2 Dosiskonzentrationen von GS-0976 untersucht. GS-0976 ist ein experimenteller, oraler Inhibitor der Acetyl-CoA-Carboxylase (ACC). Die Daten zeigen, dass die höhere GS-0976-Dosis (20 mg 1-mal täglich oral eingenommen) bei Verabreichung über 12 Wochen im Vergleich zu Placebo mit statistisch signifikanter Reduktion der hepatischen Steatose (Fettaufbau in der Leber) und einem nicht invasiven Marker der Fibrose (TIMP-1) assoziiert war. Die Studie umfasste 126 Patienten, die randomisiert 20 mg GS-0976 (n = 49), 5 mg GS-0976 (n = 51) oder Placebo (n = 26) 1-mal täglich über 12 Wochen erhielten. Bei allen Studienteilnehmern wurde NASH und Leberfibrose in den Stadien F1 bis F3 diagnostiziert, basierend auf Biopsien, Magnetresonanz-Elastographie (MRE) und Magnetresonanztomographie-Protonendichte-Fettfraktion (MRT-PDFF) [1]. Die Ergebnisse wurden auf dem internationalen Kongress «The Liver Meeting® 2017» in Washington, D.C. präsentiert (Abstract LB-9) [1]. Weitere 18 Abstracts aus der Forschungspipeline von Gilead zu NASH und Leberfibrose wurden vorgestellt.

### Literatur

1 Loomba R et al.: Acetyl-CoA carboxylase (ACC) inhibitor GS-0976 leads to significant improvements in MRI-PDFF in a phase 2, randomized, placebo-controlled trial of patients with NASH. AASLD 2017;abstr LB-9.

Gilead Sciences GmbH
*www.gilead.com*

KARGER

Fax + 49 761 4 52 07 14
Information@Karger.com
www.karger.com

*39. Münchener Fachpresse-Workshop*

## Neue Aspekte im Management gastrointestinaler Tumoren, edukative Webanwendung für NET

*Beim Management des metastasierten kolorektalen Karzinoms (mCRC) stehen laut PD Dr. Dominik P. Modest, München, derzeit die Aspekte Interdisziplinarität, Sequenztherapie und personalisierte Therapie im Mittelpunkt des Interesses.*

### *mCRC: Trifluridin/Tipiracil als Option für spätere Therapielinien*

Wie Modest erklärte, besteht beim mCRC ein großer Bedarf an Medikamenten für Therapien jenseits der Zweitlinie, denn «es gibt viele Patienten, die nach etlichen Therapien noch in gutem Allgemeinzustand und motiviert sind». Für diese Situation steht in Deutschland nur Trifluridin/Tipiracil (Lonsurf®) als evidenzbasierte und leitliniengerechte Lastline-Option zur Verfügung. In der RECOURSE-Studie konnte für das orale Zytostatikum ein signifikanter Überlebensvorteil gegenüber Placebo aufgezeigt werden [1]. «Eine Hazard-Ratio von 0,68 gegenüber Placebo in der Lastline ist attraktiv», kommentierte der Experte. Obwohl es sich bei RECOURSE um eine Lastline-Studie handelte, hätten 42% der Patienten anschließend noch eine weitere Therapie bekommen. Das zeige auch, wie dringend weitere Therapiemöglichkeiten beim mCRC gebraucht würden. Große Hoffnung wird aktuell in die molekulare Stratifizierung kolorektaler Karzinome und eine entsprechende Biomarker-orientierte Therapie gesetzt. Mittlerweile sind gegen mehrere molekular definierte Subgruppen experimentelle Lastline-Therapien verfügbar.

### *Therapiefortschritte beim metastasierten Pankreaskarzinom*

Prof. Dr. Helmut Oettle, Friedrichshafen präsentierte einen auf aktuellen Studiendaten beruhenden Algorithmus für die Sequenztherapie des metastasierten Pankreaskarzinoms, in dem die verfügbaren Erstlinientherapien dem Allgemeinzustand des Patienten entsprechend empfohlen werden. Für Patienten mit gutem Allgemeinzustand (Karnofsky Performance Status (KPS) 90–100%) stünden nab-Paclitaxel (Abraxane®) + Gemcitabin und das toxischere FOLFIRINOX zur Verfügung. Bei eingeschränktem Allgemeinzustand (KPS > 60%) sei nab-Paclitaxel + Gemcitabin die Therapie der Wahl. Patienten mit schlechtem Allgemeinzustand (KPS 50–60%) sollten eine Gemcitabin-Monotherapie erhalten, so Oettle.
Die Phase-III-Studie MPACT, die bei unbehandelten Patienten mit metastasiertem Pankreaskarzinom nab-Paclitaxel + Gemcitabin mit Gemcitabin alleine verglich, hatte einen Überlebensvorteil für nab-Paclitaxel + Gemcitabin gezeigt [2]. Aktuell wird diese Kombination in der Phase-II-Studie LAPACT für die lokal fortgeschrittene Situation geprüft. Die beim Kongress der European Society for Medical Oncology (ESMO) 2017 vorgestellten Interimsdaten ergaben eine Krankheitskontrollrate von 82% und eine Remissionsrate von 35% [3]. Eine Real-Life-Studie an deutschen Zentren zeigte, dass die Überlebenschancen stark mit dem Allgemeinzustand korrelierten und dass die Neurotoxizität von nab-Paclitaxel + Gemcitabin im Praxisalltag eine geringere Rolle spielte als vermutet [4].

### *Mit net-Xpert Diagnostik und Therapie von NET trainieren*

Dr. Alexander König, Göttingen, stellte die in Kooperation mit Novartis Oncology entwickelte neue Webanwendung net-Xpert vor, die Ärzten die Möglichkeit gibt, anhand verschiedener realer Patientenfälle im praxisnahen Training ihr Wissen über die Diagnose und Therapie von neuroendokrinen Tumoren (NET) zu vertiefen. NET sind eine seltene Tumorentität, deren Häufigkeit in den letzten Jahren sprunghaft angestiegen ist. Bei G1-Tumoren mit einer niedrigen Proliferationsrate (Ki-67 ≤ 2%) beträgt das mittlere Gesamtüberleben etwa 10 Jahre. Bei NET G2-Tumoren (Ki-67-Wert 3–20%) liegt es bei etwa 5 Jahren, bei NET G3-Tumoren (Ki-67 > 20%) bei 15 Monaten. Mittlerweile stehen verschiedene Therapieoptionen zur Verfügung. net-Xpert ist ein Algorithmentraining, das auf realen Fällen beruht. Jeder Fall in net-Xpert dient dabei dem Erlernen bzw. Vertiefen eines Teilaspekts in der Diagnostik oder Behandlung. Nach Abschluss eines Falls kann der Anwender durch Bearbeitung eines Fragenkatalogs CME-Punkte (CME = Continuing Medical Education) erwerben. net-Xpert steht als Web-Anwendung für den PC und als App für Mobilgeräte zur Verfügung.

*Andrea Schäffer, Holzkirchen*

### *Quelle*

39. Münchener Fachpresse-Workshop der POMME-med GmbH, 17. Oktober 2017, München; Gemeinsame Sponsoren: Celgene GmbH, Mundipharma GmbH & Co. KG, Novartis Pharma GmbH, Servier Deutschland GmbH, Tesaro Bio Germany GmbH

### *Literatur*

1 Mayer RJ et al.: N Engl J Med 2015;372:1909–1919.
2 Von Hoff DD et al.: N Engl J Med 2013;369:1691–1703.
3 Philip AP et al.: Ann Oncol 2017;28(suppl 5):v209–v268.
4 Al-Batran SE et al.: ESMO 2017;abstr 751P.

Weitere Informationen bei
POMME-med GmbH
*www.pomme-med.de*

## Ein Jahr ONIVYDE – Wie hat sich die Therapie für Patienten mit metastasiertem Pankreaskarzinom verändert?

ONIVYDE (pegyliertes liposomales Irinotecan, nal-IRI) in Kombination mit 5-Fluorouracil (5-FU) und Leucovorin (LV) ist das bisher einzige zugelassene Medikament für die Behandlung von Patienten mit metastasiertem Adenokarzinom des Pankreas, deren Erkrankung unter einer Gemcitabin-basierten Therapie fortgeschritten ist (post-Gemcitabin) [1]. «Liposomal verkapseltes Irinotecan (nal-IRI) ist gut einsetzbar, und der Behandlungsalltag spiegelt die Datenlage wider: Patienten profitieren sowohl nach Vorbehandlung mit einer Gemcitabin-Kombinationstherapie als auch mit Gemcitabin-Monotherapie von dem nal-IRI-haltigen Regime und können nun eine weitere Therapielinie angeboten bekommen», erklärt Prof. Manfred P. Lutz, Chefarzt der Medizinischen Klinik am Caritas-Klinikum Saarbrücken St. Theresia, auf einer Fachpresseveranstaltung während der Jahrestagung der Deutschen, Österreichischen und Schweizerischen Gesellschaften für Hämatologie und Medizinische Onkologie vom 29.09. bis 03.10.2017 in Stuttgart. Für die Behandlung des metastasierten Pankreaskarzinoms ist eine Gemcitabin-haltige Therapie Standard. Noch bis vor einem Jahr stand keine zugelassene Behandlungsoption für den Fall, dass die Gemcitabin-haltige Therapie versagt hat, zur Verfügung. Dies hat sich mit der Zulassung von ONIVYDE grundlegend geändert.
Im Rahmen einer Preisverleihung am 19. Oktober 2017 in Berlin wurde der diesjährige Galenus-von-Pergamon-Preis verliehen, bei der ONIVYDE das Finale in der Kategorie «Orphan Drugs» erreichte.

### *Literatur*

1 Fachinformation ONIVYDE, Stand Oktober 2016.

Shire Deutschland GmbH
*www.shire.de*

KARGER

Fax + 49 761 4 52 07 14
Information@Karger.com
www.karger.com

Visc Med 33 | 6 | 17

*Karzinoidsyndrom-bedingte Diarrhö*

## Add-on-Therapie mit Telotristatethyl erhöht Lebensqualität deutlich

*Bei Patienten mit neuroendokrinen Tumoren (NET) kann durch eine Serotonin-Hypersekretion ein Karzinoidsyndrom entstehen, das sich unter anderem durch sekretorische Diarrhö auszeichnet. Die Add-on-Therapie mit Telotristatethyl senkt die tägliche Stuhlfrequenz deutlich und verbessert somit bei günstigem Sicherheitsprofil die Lebensqualität.*

Beim Karzinoidsyndrom besteht ein hoher Krankheitsdruck, da die Symptome mit einer reduzierten Lebensqualität assoziiert sind. «Vor allem Durchfall und zu häufiger bzw. dringender Stuhlgang werden als besonders belastend empfunden», berichtete Prof. Dieter Hörsch, Bad Berka. Die Diarrhö geht auf Serotonin zurück, das vom Tumor produziert wird. Die erste Wahl bei der Behandlung sind Somatostatin-Analoga (SSA). Kann unter der SSA-Behandlung keine ausreichende Symptomkontrolle erzielt werden, ist zur Therapie der Karzinoidsyndrom-bedingten Diarrhö in Kombination mit einem SSA Telotristatethyl (Xermelo®) indiziert. Während SSA lediglich die Serotonin-Sekretion verhindern, blockiert der erste und einzige zugelassene, orale Tryptophan-Hydroxylase-Inhibitor die Biosynthese von Serotonin, indem die Tryptophan-Hydroxylase und die aromatische L-Aminosäure-Decarboxylase in der NET-Zelle gehemmt werden, entschlüsselte Prof. Marianne Pavel, Erlangen, den Wirkmechanismus. Dabei passiert der Wirkstoff nicht die Blut-Hirn-Schranke.

### *Studien belegen Wirksamkeit und Sicherheit*

Die Ergebnisse der Phase-III-Studien TELESTAR [1] und TELECAST [2] belegen Wirksamkeit und Sicherheit: Das arithmetische Mittel der Reduktion der täglichen Stuhlfrequenz in Woche 12 gegenüber Baseline lag für Telotristatethyl bei –1,7 (250 mg) bzw. –2,1 (500 mg) im Vergleich zu –0,9 im Placeboarm, dokumentierte Pavel nach den Ergebnissen der Studie TELESTAR. Ein anhaltendes Ansprechen wurde bei 44% (250 mg) bzw. 42% (500 mg) der Patienten beobachtet versus 20% unter Placebo. Die Menge des Serotonin-Metaboliten 5-Hydroxyindolessigsäure (5-HIES) im 24-Stunden-Urin war mit –40,1 mg (250 mg) bzw. –57,7 mg (500 mg) signifikant reduziert, während sie unter Placebo um 11,5 mg anstieg.

Diese Ergebnisse spiegeln sich auch in der Verbesserung der Lebensqualität wider: 56% der Patienten waren unter Telotristatethyl plus SSA sehr zufrieden mit ihrer Behandlung versus 0% unter Placebo. Es wurde eine allgemein gute Verträglichkeit beobachtet. Telotristatethyl zeichnete sich durch ein günstiges Sicherheitsprofil aus und es wurde kein Sicherheitssignal berichtet, dass Depressionen auftreten. Zum Zeitpunkt des Ausscheidens aus der Studie gaben 88% der Patienten bei einer Befragung an, dass sich die Symptome verbessert haben. Von diesen berichteten 95% eine bedeutsame Reduktion der Stuhlfrequenz.

Auch in der Begleitstudie TELECAST, die ähnlich aufgebaut war, wurden die beiden primären Endpunkte, Verträglichkeit und 5-HIES-Reduktion, erreicht, so Pavel: Während in der Placebogruppe kein Patient ansprach, wurde unter Telotristatethyl bei 40% der Patienten eine Reduktion der Stuhlfrequenz von mindestens 30% festgestellt. Die prozentuale Veränderung der 5-HIES-Ausscheidung betrug –33,2% (250 mg) bzw. –76,5% (500 mg) unter Verum versus +97,7% in der Placebogruppe. Die gute Verträglichkeit war konsistent zu den Daten der TELESTAR-Studie. Studienabbrüche aufgrund von Depression oder erhöhter Leberwerte traten nicht auf.

«Telotristatethyl bietet in der Behandlung des Karzinoidsyndroms eine sehr gute neue Möglichkeit bei klinisch guter Verträglichkeit», fasste Hörsch die klinischen Erfahrungen zusammen.

*Sabine M. Rüdesheim, Frechen*

*Quelle*

Launch-Presseveranstaltung «Xermelo® (Telotristatethyl) – mehr Über-Lebensqualität für Menschen mit Karzinoid-Syndrom-bedingter Diarrhö», 18.10.2017, Frankfurt, Veranstalter: Ipsen Pharma

*Literatur*

1 Kulke M et al.: J Clin Oncol 2017;35:14–23.
2 Pavel M et al.: NANETS 2016;abstr C8.

Weitere Informationen bei
Ipsen Pharma GmbH
*www.ipsen.com*

## Neue Daten zu Ramucirumab vom ESMO-Kongress 2017 – Gute Verträglichkeit unabhängig von Therapieregime und Tumorentität

Seit Anfang 2016 ist der Angiogenesehemmer Ramucirumab (CYRAMZA®) in Kombination mit FOLFIRI EU-weit für die Zweitlinientherapie von Patienten mit metastasiertem Kolorektalkarzinom (mCRC) zugelassen [1]. Aus einer kürzlich auf dem ESMO-Kongress vorgestellten Analyse der Zulassungsstudie RAISE gibt es jetzt einen ersten Hinweis auf einen möglichen prädiktiven Biomarker für die Effektivität von Ramucirumab [2]: Ein höherer Spiegel an VEGF-D im Blutplasma war in der Studie mit einer Verlängerung von progressionsfreiem Überleben und Gesamtüberleben durch die Ramucirumab-haltige Therapie assoziiert. Präsentiert wurde auch eine Metaanalyse von Ramucirumab-Studien, die das gute Verträglichkeitsprofil der Substanz untermauert [3].
In der Phase-3-Studie RAISE an 1072 mit Bevacizumab und Oxaliplatin vorbehandelten mCRC-Patienten hatte das Regime mit Ramucirumab plus FOLFIRI den primären Endpunkt Gesamtüberleben im Vergleich zu FOLFIRI allein signifikant verlängert (13,3 vs. 11,7 Monate; Hazard Ratio (HR) 0,844; p = 0,0219) [4]. «Das Gesamtüberleben ist in der Zweitliniensituation ein sehr harter Endpunkt» betonte Prof. Dr. Dirk Arnold, Hamburg und Lissabon, auf einem Presse-Talk am Rande des ESMO-Kongresses [5].

*Literatur*

1 Fachinformation CYRAMZA®, Stand: Januar 2016.
2 Tabernero J et al.: ESMO 2017;abstr 555P.
3 Arnold D et al.: ESMO 2017;abstr 1592P.
4 Tabernero J et al.: Lancet Oncol 2015;16:499–508.
5 Media Lunch Talk von Lilly Oncology «ESMO 2017 Madrid», 11. September 2017.

Lilly Deutschland GmbH
*www.lilly-pharma.de*

KARGER

Fax + 49 761 4 52 07 14
Information@Karger.com
www.karger.com

Visc Med 33 | 6 | 17

## Positives Ergebnis der klinischen Phase-III-Studie zur Induktionstherapie mit Mesalazin bei Colitis ulcerosa veröffentlicht

Kürzlich wurden die vollständigen Ergebnisse der Phase-III-Non-Inferiority-Studie zur Behandlung leichter bis mäßig aktiver Colitis ulcerosa (CU) mit 1600-mg-Mesalazin-Tabletten im Vergleich zu 400-mg-Mesalazin-Tabletten in der Fachzeitschrift ALIMENTARY PHARMACOLOGY & THERAPEUTICS veröffentlicht [1]. In Europa leiden bis zu 3 Millionen Menschen an entzündlichen Darmerkrankungen wie CU [2]. Ziel der von Tillotts Pharma AG durchgeführten Doppelblind-Studie war es, die Wirksamkeit und Sicherheit einer neu entwickelten 1600-mg-Mesalazin-Formulierung mit der 400-mg-Tablette zu vergleichen. Die Untersuchungsergebnisse zeigen, dass das primäre Studienziel erreicht wurde [1].

Unter der Leitung von Prof. Dr. Geert D'Haens nahmen mehr als 800 Patientinnen und Patienten in rund 180 Zentren in Europa und Kanada an der Studie teil. Es handelt sich damit um die vermutlich umfangreichste Studie zur Akutbehandlung leichter bis mäßig aktiver CU mit Mesalazin [1]. Die Patientinnen und Patienten wurden nach dem Zufallsprinzip in zwei Gruppen eingeteilt und erhielten 3,2 g Mesalazin oral verabreicht. Sie nahmen 1-mal täglich zwei 1600-mg-Tabletten oder 2-mal täglich vier 400-mg-Tabletten ein. Die Ärzte, die zentralen Auswerter sowie die Patientinnen und Patienten wussten nicht, welcher Behandlungsgruppe sie zugeordnet worden waren. In der Studie wurde die Therapie von einem zentralen, unabhängigen Auswerter anhand einer anonymisierten endoskopischen Videobeurteilung untersucht [1]. Die Einschlusskriterien der Studie und die unvoreingenommene Interpretation des endoskopischen Bildmaterials werden damit strikt eingehalten [2, 3]. Eine unabhängige Beurteilung der Bilder wird durch die Regulierungsbehörden verlangt und bei Phase-III-Studien zu CU als unverzichtbar angesehen [2].

### *Literatur*


1 D'Haens GR et al.: Aliment Pharmacol Ther 2017;46:292–302.
2 Kaplan G: Nat Rev Gastroenterol Hepatol 2015;12:720–727.
3 Gottlieb K et al.: Inflamm Bowel Dis 2015;21:2475–2482.


Weitere Informationen bei
Tillotts Pharma GmbH
*www.tillotts.com*

## Schmerztherapie erleichtern – durch kausale Behandlung der Opioid-induzierten Obstipation (OIC)

Opioid-Analgetika sind für die Behandlung chronischer Schmerzen essenziell [1]. Sie vermitteln ihre schmerzlindernde Wirkung über µ-Opioid-Rezeptoren im zentralen Nervensystem (ZNS); im Gastrointestinaltrakt hingegen kann ihre agonistische Wirkung auf µ-Opioid-Rezeptoren zur häufigsten Nebenwirkung der Opioid-Therapie führen, der Opioid-induzierten Obstipation (OIC) [2]. Unbehandelt kann die OIC die Gesamtlast der Erkrankung bei Schmerzpatienten erhöhen [3]. Aufgrund der Pathogenese der OIC sind weder Erstmaßnahmen wie Flüssigkeitsaufnahme und Ballaststoffe hilfreich, auch führen Laxanzien oftmals zu keiner Linderung der Beschwerden [4, 5]. Bei unzureichendem Ansprechen auf Laxanzien kann der kausale Wirkansatz von peripher wirkenden µ-Opioid-Rezeptor-Antagonisten (PAMORA) wie Naloxegol (Moventig®) zur effektiven Behandlung der OIC beitragen [6] und eine dosisgerechte Durchführung der Schmerztherapie gewährleisten, wie PD Dr. Stefan Wirz, Bad Honnef, in einem Interview berichtet.

Eine OIC kann jederzeit nach Einleitung einer Opioid-Therapie und bereits bei Verwendung schwacher Opioid-Analgetika und bei niedrigen Dosierungen auftreten [7, 8].

Die Folge ist das Auftreten von zum Beispiel hartem Stuhlgang und mühevoller, oft inkompletter Stuhlentleerung sowie begleitend auftretendes Völlegefühl, Bauchdruck und -schmerzen, Blähungen, Übelkeit und Erbrechen [9–11]. Die Lebensqualität von Patienten mit OIC ist erheblich verringert [12]. Jeder vierte mit Laxanzien versorgte Schmerzpatient versucht, die OIC-Symptomatik zu reduzieren, indem er die Opioid-Dosis verringert oder das Opioid seltener einnimmt [13]. Oft wird ganz auf das Opioid verzichtet, denn die bestehenden Schmerzen können erträglicher sein als die Nebenwirkungen der Opioid-Therapie [13, 14]. Bereits zu Beginn einer Opioid-Therapie kann eine Stratifizierung des Obstipationsrisikos helfen, um ihren Effekt auf den Stuhlgang einzuschätzen. Dr. Wirz rät, hierzu den Allgemeinzustand, den Mobilitäts- und Flüssigkeitsstatus eines Patienten sowie die bereits bestehende Einnahme obstipationsfördernder Medikamente zu berücksichtigen. Zu Beginn der Opioid-Therapie können prophylaktisch Laxanzien verschrieben werden [15]. Die OIC-Symptome persistieren unter einer Laxanzien-Therapie bei mehr als der Hälfte der Patienten, wie Untersuchungen zeigen [9, 10]. Bei geringem Ansprechen oder Versagen sollte deshalb eine kausale Therapie mit PAMORA zum Einsatz kommen, da sie auf die wesentlichen Mechanismen der OIC – die Hemmung des peristaltischen Reflexes und der gastrointestinalen Sekretion – abzielt [11].

Der erste oral verfügbare Vertreter der PAMORA ist Naloxegol, ein pegyliertes Derivat des µ-Opioid-Rezeptor-Antagonisten Naloxon [6]. Die Wirksamkeit und Sicherheit der Behandlung mit Naloxegol wurde in den randomisierten placebokontrollierten Phase-III-Studien KODIAC 4 und KODIAC 5 evaluiert [16, 17]. «Naloxegol kann in Bezug auf das eingesetzte Opioid viel einfacher und unkomplizierter angewendet werden als das unspezifische Naloxon», sagte Dr. Wirz im Interview. «Man muss das Verhältnis zwischen Agonist und Antagonist nicht austarieren. Aufgrund seiner Pegylierung überwindet Naloxegol die Blut-Hirn-Schranke nicht in klinischem Maße. Die gewünschte analgetische Wirkung der Opioid-Therapie bleibt damit erhalten. Zudem kann der PAMORA die µ-Rezeptoraktivität verschiedener Opioide antagonisieren und ist daher einfach und breit einsetzbar.»

### *Literatur*


1 Häuser W et al.: Dtsch Arztebl 2014;111:732–740.
2 Yoon SC, Bruner HC: Patient Prefer Adherence 2017;11:1265–1271.
3 Bell TJ et al.: Pain Med 2009;10:35–42.
4 Kumar L et al.: Gastroenterol Res Pract 2014;2014:141737.
5 Palmer CS et al.: 20th Annual Scientific Meeting of the American Pain Society, Phoenix/Arizona, USA, 19.–22. April 2001;abstr 790.
6 Fachinformation Moventig®, Stand September 2016.
7 Nelson AD, Camilleri M: Ther Adv Chronic Dis 2016;7:121–134.
8 Lawson R et al.: Adv Ther 2016;33:1331–1346.
9 Coyne KS et al.: Front Oncol 2016;6:131.
10 Pappagallo M: Am J Surg 2001;182(suppl 5A):11S–18S.
11 Andresen V, Wedel T: Arzneiverordnung in der Praxis 2016;43(1).
12 Siemens W et al.: Expert Opin Pharmacother 2014;16:515–532.
13 Petersen K-U: Verdauungskrankheiten 2016;34:244–257.
14 Lawson R et al.: Adv Ther 2016;33:1331–1346.
15 Andresen V et al.: Z Gastroenterol 2013;51:651–672.
16 Chey WD et al.: N Engl J Med 2014;370:2387–2396.
17 Tack J et al.: United European Gastroenterol J 2015;3:471–480.


Weitere Informationen bei
Kyowa Kirin GmbH
*www.kyowa-kirin.com*

KARGER

Fax + 49 761 4 52 07 14
Information@Karger.com
www.karger.com

Visceral Medicine

# Meetings and Conferences

Visc Med 2017;33:483–485

| | | |
|---|---|---|
| **20.01.2018**<br>**Munich**<br>Germany | **TZM-Essentials 2018** | **Information:** www.tzm-essentials.de |
| **25.01.–27.01.2018**<br>**Ulm**<br>Germany | **38. Jahrestagung des Deutschen Pankreasclubs** | **Information:** www.dpc-kongress.de |
| **26.01.–27.01.2018**<br>**Berlin**<br>Germany | **12. Jahrestagung der Gesellschaft für Gastroenterologie und Hepatologie in Berlin und Brandenburg** | **Information:** www.gghbb.de |
| **26.01.–27.01.2018**<br>**Mannheim**<br>Germany | **24. AGIO Winterkurs der DGVS** | **Information:**<br>www.dgvs.de/fortbildung-aktuell/dgvs-veranstaltungen |
| **01.02.–03.02.2018**<br>**Düsseldorf**<br>Germany | **20. Internationales Endoskopie Symposium** | **Information:** www.endo-duesseldorf.com |
| **07.02.–09.02.2018**<br>**Kloster Drübeck**<br>Germany | **DGHO Juniorakademie 2018** | **Information:** www.dgho-service.de/veranstaltungen/dgho-juniorakademie-2018 |
| **14.02.–17.02.2018**<br>**Vienna**<br>Austria | **ECCO 2018 – European Cancer Congress** | **Information:** www.ecco-ibd.eu/ecco18 |
| **17.02.–20.02.2018**<br>**Leipzig**<br>Germany | **47. Jahrestagung der Deutschen Gesellschaft für Thorax-, Herz- und Gefäßchirurgie** | **Information:** www.dgthg-jahrestagung.de |
| **21.02.–24.02.2018**<br>**Berlin**<br>Germany | **33. Deutscher Krebskongress** | **Information:** www.dkk2018.de |
| **23.02.2018**<br>**Hamburg**<br>Germany | **Endo Club Spring** | **Information:** www.endoclubspring.de |
| **23.02.–24.02.2018**<br>**Nuremberg**<br>Germany | **Bundeskongress Chirurgie 2018** | **Information:** www.bundeskongress-chirurgie.de |
| **01.03.–03.03.2018**<br>**Neustadt/Weinstraße**<br>Germany | **62. Jahrestagung der Saarländisch-Pfälzischen Internistischen Gesellschaft** | **Information:** www.spig.org |
| **02.03.–03.03.2018**<br>**Freiburg i.Br.**<br>Germany | **European Symposium on Minimally Invasive Surgery** | **Information:** www.mis-symposium.de |
| **02.03.–03.03.2018**<br>**Mannheim**<br>Germany | **Anorektaler Endosonographiekurs** | **Information:** fuks@bkb.info |
| **02.03.–04.03.2018**<br>**Freising**<br>Germany | **25. Jahrestagung der Deutschen Gesellschaft für Neurogastroenterologie und Motilität** | **Information:** www.neurogastro.de |
| **08.03.–10.03.2018**<br>**Mannheim**<br>Germany | **19. DGVS-Seminar Chronisch entzündliche Darmerkrankungen – Modul 1** | **Information:**<br>www.dgvs.de/fortbildung-aktuell/dgvs-veranstaltungen |

KARGER
Fax +49 761 4 52 07 14
Information@Karger.com
www.karger.com



Accessible online at:
www.karger.com/vis

| | | |
|---|---|---|
| **15.03.–17.03.2018**<br>**Mannheim**<br>Germany | **21. DGVS-Seminar Onkologische Gastroenterologie – Modul 1** | **Information:** www.dgvs.de/fortbildung-aktuell/dgvs-veranstaltungen |
| **15.03.–17.03.2018**<br>**St. Gallen**<br>Switzerland | **4th International Gastrointestinal Cancer Conference – Primary Therapy of Early GI Cancer** | **Information:** www.oncoconferences.ch |
| **15.03.–17.03.2018**<br>**Munich**<br>Germany | **48. Kongress der Deutschen Gesellschaft für Endoskopie und Bildgebende Verfahren** | **Information:** www.dge-bv.de |
| **15.03.–17.03.2018**<br>**Munich**<br>Germany | **44. Deutscher Koloproktologen-Kongress** | **Information:** www.koloproktologen-kongress.de |
| **14.04.–17.04.2018**<br>**Mannheim**<br>Germany | **124. Kongress der Deutschen Gesellschaft für Innere Medizin (DGIM)** | **Information:** www.dgim.de |
| **17.04.–20.04.2018**<br>**Berlin**<br>Germany | **135. Kongress der Deutschen Gesellschaft für Chirurgie** | **Information:** www.chirurgie2018.de |
| **20.04.–21.04.2018**<br>**Berlin**<br>Germany | **12. AIO-GI-Tag** | **Information:** aio@krebsgesellschaft.de |
| **27.04.–28.04.2018**<br>**Berlin**<br>Germany | **Endoskopie Live 2018** | **Information:** www.endoskopie-live-berlin.de |
| **27.04.–28.04.2018**<br>**Berlin**<br>Germany | **7. Hepatologie-Update-Seminar** | **Information:** www.hepato-update.com |
| **31.05.–02.06.2018**<br>**Leipzig**<br>Germany | **1. Gemeinsame Jahrestagung der Mitteldeutschen Chirurgenvereinigung und der Mitteldeutschen Gesellschaft für Gastroenterologie** | **Information:** www.mgfg.de |
| **06.06.–08.06.2018**<br>**Vienna**<br>Austria | **59. Österreichischer Chirurgenkongress** | **Information:** www.chirurgenkongress.at |
| **07.06.–08.06.2018**<br>**Dortmund**<br>Germany | **Viszeralmedizin NRW 2018** | **Information:** www.viszeralmedizin-nrw.de |
| **08.06.–09.06.2018**<br>**Ludwigshafen**<br>Germany | **6. Ludwigshafener GastroTage** | **Information:** www.gastrotagelu.de |
| **09.06.2018**<br>**Wiesbaden**<br>Germany | **14. Interdisziplinäres GI-Oncology Update** | **Information:** www.gi-oncology.de |
| **14.06.–15.06.2018**<br>**Munich**<br>Germany | **46. Jahrestagung der Gesellschaft für Gastroenterologie in Bayern** | **Information:** www.gfgb.org |
| **14.06.–16.06.2018**<br>**Salzburg**<br>Austria | **51. Jahrestagung und 29. Fortbildungskurs der Österreichischen Gesellschaft für Gastroenterologie und Hepatologie** | **Information:** www.oeggh.at/veranstaltungen |
| **20.06.–23.06.2018**<br>**Cologne**<br>Germany | **KIT 2018 – Kongress für Infektionskrankheiten und Tropenmedizin** | **Information:** www.kit2018.de |
| **21.06.–23.06.2018**<br>**Kassel**<br>Germany | **Ernährung 2018 – Ernährung ist Therapie und Prävention** | **Information:** www.ernaehrung2018.de |
| **29.06.–30.06.2018**<br>**Hanover**<br>Germany | **15. HepNet Symposium** | **Information:** www.deutsche-leberstiftung.de/symposium |

| | | |
|---|---|---|
| **30.06.2018**<br>**Wiesbaden**<br>Germany | **GI-Oncology – 14. Interdisziplinäres Update** | **Information:** www.gi-oncology.de |
| **18.07.–20.07.2018**<br>**Garmisch-Partenkirchen**<br>Germany | **95. Jahrestagung der Vereinigung Bayerischer Chirurgen (VBC) – Ganzheitliche Chirurgie** | **Information:** www.www.vbc2018.de.de |
| **12.09.–15.09.2018**<br>**Munich**<br>Germany | **Viszeralmedizin 2018** | **Information:** www.viszeralmedizin.com |
| **28.09.–02.10.2018**<br>**Vienna**<br>Austria | **Jahrestagung der Deutschen, Österreichischen und Schweizerischen Gesellschaften für Hämatologie und Medizinische Onkologie** | **Information:** www.haematologie-onkologie-2018.com |
| **02.11.–03.11.2018**<br>**Hamburg**<br>Germany | **Endo Club Nord 2018** | **Information:** www.endoclubnord.de |
| **08.11.–10.11.2018**<br>**Mannheim**<br>Germany | **21. DGVS-Seminar Onkologische Gastroenterologie – Modul 2** | **Information:**<br>www.dgvs.de/fortbildung-aktuell/dgvs-veranstaltungen |
| **15.11.–17.11.2018**<br>**Mannheim**<br>Germany | **19. DGVS-Seminar Chronisch entzündliche Darmerkrankungen – Modul 2** | **Information:**<br>www.dgvs.de/fortbildung-aktuell/dgvs-veranstaltungen |
| **05.12.–08.12.2018**<br>**Berlin**<br>Germany | **17. DGVS-Seminar Hepatologie – Modul 1** | **Information:**<br>www.dgvs.de/fortbildung-aktuell/dgvs-veranstaltungen |
| **06.03.–09.03.2019**<br>**Berlin**<br>Germany | **17. DGVS-Seminar Hepatologie – Modul 20** | **Information:**<br>www.dgvs.de/fortbildung-aktuell/dgvs-veranstaltungen |

Visceral Medicine

# Contents Vol. 33, 2017

Visc Med 2017;33:486–488

## Focuses



## Editorials



## Clinical Therapeutic Review



## Interdisciplinary Discussion



## Original Article



KARGER
Fax +49 761 4 52 07 14
Information@Karger.com
www.karger.com



Accessible online at:
www.karger.com/vim

**Review Articles**